TONY CHRISTIANSEN'S SECRETS OF SUCCESS

ATTITUDE PLUS!

TONY CHRISTIANSEN'S
SECRETS OF SUCCESS

ATTITUDE PLUS!

TONY CHRISTIANSEN
with Liz McKeown

HarperCollinsPublishers

National Library of New Zealand Cataloguing-in-Publication Data

Christiansen, Tony.
Attitude plus! : Tony Christiansen's secret of success / Tony Christiansen and Liz McKeown.
ISBN 1-86950-470-4
1. Christiansen, Tony. 2. Self-actualization (Psychology)
3. Success. 4. Amputees—New Zealand—Biography.
I. McKeown, Liz. II. Title.
158.1—dc 21

First published 2003
HarperCollins*Publishers* (New Zealand) Limited
P.O. Box 1, Auckland

Copyright © Tony Christiansen 2003

Tony Christiansen and Liz McKeown assert the moral right
to be identified as the authors of this work.

All rights reserved. No part of this publication may be reproduced
or stored in a retrieval system or transmitted in any form or by
any means, electronic, mechanical, photocopying, recording or
otherwise, without the prior written permission of the publishers.

ISBN 1 86950 470 4

Front cover photo by Chris Parker Photografix, Tauranga
Back cover photos by KBS (Korean Broadcasting Service)
Set in Cheltenham 9.5 pt
Printed by Griffin Press, Australia

contents

	Preface	7
1	Bigger and Better	9
2	Making a Difference	20
3	Perceptions and Misconceptions	40
4	A Wealth of Choices	60
5	The Power of Positive Thinking	81
6	The Risk Factor	101
7	Off to Africa	119
8	The Crown of Africa	140
9	More Mountains to Climb	157

preface

The volcanic massif of Kilimanjaro rises straight out of the plain in northern Tanzania, and its bulk extends some 80 kilometres from east to west. Its highest point, Uhuru Peak, is the 'Crown of Africa'. At 5895 metres high, the mountain's upper levels are very cold, the oxygen thins out, and the weather can deteriorate rapidly to freezing sleet, wind and snow. Kilimanjaro means 'unclimbable mountain', but that hasn't stopped scores of people making it to the top of Africa's highest peak, and today ascents are carefully controlled commercial operations, although the climb remains a formidable challenge to anyone.

In December 2002 a motley team of people formed an odd group on the mountain's slopes. They included Soo Young, a blind Korean woman in her thirties, Hong Bin, a Korean climber who had lost the fingers on both his hands to frostbite, assorted New Zealand and Korean climbers, minders and documentary makers, and African guides and porters. And me, Tony Christiansen, from Tauranga, New Zealand, with no legs, in a wheelchair.

What on earth was I doing there? Climbing Kilimanjaro, of course! Although, I have to admit, at certain points on the way up I did wonder why – but not for long. The exhilaration and sense of accomplishment I was soon to feel would banish any doubts.

Actually, it has usually been other people who have held doubts on my behalf. Before leaving New Zealand for the climb, numerous people told me I was crazy for even contemplating such a feat. Others said I'd never be able to do it and that I shouldn't even be trying. Best friends suggested I was 'bloody mad'.

It was a long way from losing my legs as a nine-year-old in Tauranga to climbing Kilimanjaro, and I have told some of the story of my life and experiences in my first book, *Race You to the Top*. The opening part of this book recaps briefly some of what happened in my life, what I made happen in my life, and what led me to finally be on the mountain just before Christmas 2002, with a strange assortment of fellow travellers.

After listening to the warnings about climbing Kilimanjaro, the advice and questioning of my sanity, I reached the conclusion that some would say these things because they would never dream of doing such a climb themselves. Perhaps they didn't like to see me taking risks they weren't prepared to take themselves. Perhaps they were envious. I've had people tell me I make them feel inadequate, but that is certainly not my intention. Some say it is all about ego and one-upmanship, that I'm trying to prove I'm better than everybody else. But it is not like that at all. I do the things I do because I want to, because I enjoy doing them and because I have the opportunities to do them.

In *Attitude Plus!* I want to share some of what and who has inspired me, motivated me and helped me achieve what I have wanted to do. I'm an uncomplicated person and my messages are straightforward, simple and commonsensical. In the second part of the book, I relate stories and experiences from which I draw some key messages, which I hope will challenge and provoke you, and hopefully assist you to meet your challenges.

In the last chapters of the book, we're off to Africa. During the day, Kilimanjaro is usually obscured by cloud, lending it an air of mystery, but in the clear dawn light, in a town not far from its feet, I got my first glimpse of the mountain. It was beautiful, massive and quite forbidding. At the moment I saw it, though, I knew I would climb it. I said to myself, 'This is what we came here for and this is what I'm going to do.' And I did.

I hope you get to do the things you want, and that you have fun doing them.

Best wishes
Tony Christiansen

bigger and better | 1

We're here for a good time, not a long time.

It is three years since I wrote my first book, *Race You to the Top*, and I've been overwhelmed by the interest it has created not just in my home country, New Zealand, but in many other parts of the world too. Many of those who've bought it have been people who have attended one of my speaking presentations in countries such as Australia, South Africa, Thailand, Canada and the United States. The book is currently being translated into Korean because I've become something of a celebrity there thanks to a couple of documentaries I've featured in on Korean television.

The title *Race You to the Top* was a play on the fact that I have always been passionate about motor racing and I always strive to be the best at whatever I undertake, or at least to do the best that I can. In other words, I aim for the top. Never in my wildest dreams did I think the title would assume a new significance when, less than three years later, I found myself on top of the highest mountain in Africa, Mt Kilimanjaro. But I guess that's the story of my life. I never know from one day to the next what opportunities are going to present themselves, what choices I'm going to have to make and what risks might be involved. I have always been adventurous and ambitious, but even I find it hard to believe just how much my life has changed in recent years.

In 2000 I was just embarking on a new career as a professional inspirational speaker after having been a signwriter for most of my life. It was a fairly dramatic change, although one thing stayed the same. I was used to shinning up trestles to paint my signs and it was a practice that never failed to impress onlookers, so I decided to incorporate it into my presentation. Having no legs means I'm somewhat vertically challenged and as I don't like wearing artificial legs I can be a bit hard to see standing behind a podium. And I never, ever speak from my wheelchair because when people see you in a wheelchair they see only your supposed *disability*. That's their perception thanks to the world we've been brought up in. But I need my audience to see the abilities I have rather than the perceived disabilities. So I wheel myself up to the trestles in my chair, climb up the framework and then deliver my speech from a plank of wood a couple of metres off the ground. It certainly sets me apart from other inspirational speakers and it is one way of getting everyone's attention. Those watching are too scared to take their eyes off me in case I fall off my plank!

Actually, I soon discovered that being a good professional speaker means you have to be a good entertainer as well. You can't just stand up on stage, rattle off a lot of wise words and expect everyone to stay riveted and awake. You've got to get up there and sock it to them with passion and pizzazz, and that's something I really enjoy.

It is a bit like being an actor. I have to constantly come up with new ways of getting my message across and I guess I'm lucky that in this technological age there are all sorts of computerised techniques to add a new dimension. I'm able to flash illustrations, quotations and video clips of some of my sporting achievements onto big screens and I've also had three songs especially written for me by Australian musician and singer Martin Way. He's included them on a CD called *Inside Out* and I think he's done a great job capturing the essence of my message with his music and lyrics.

Right from the start of my career as a professional speaker I've made a point of staying at the back of the hall, out of sight, while my credentials are read out to the audience. When people are told that the next speaker flies planes, races cars, has a black belt in tae kwon do and is a champion surf lifesaver they form an image of a strong, six-foot tall, broad-shouldered and bronzed young Adonis. Instead they get me zooming down the aisle in my wheelchair, no legs and very little hair — but masses of energy. Oh, and yes, I do have broad shoulders. So they've already learnt lesson number one before I've even opened my mouth: don't judge a book by its cover.

Obviously, it took a while for me to become well known on the speaking circuit, but it is amazing how quickly things can happen if you put in the effort and have the enthusiasm. The first year after I swapped signwriting for speaking I only had about 50 engagements. That nearly doubled the second year and now every week I find myself on a plane bound for yet another destination: Bangkok, Dubai, Toronto, New York, Miami, Nashville, Fiji, Vanuatu, Singapore, Sydney, Surfers Paradise — I've been to them all and more in the past three years. I've met all kinds of interesting people and stayed in all the best hotels and loved every minute of it.

As a young athlete I'd travelled overseas quite a few times but I always flew economy class on package deals that saw me accommodated in cheap hotels or hostels. These days I tend to stay somewhere posh like the Hilton, the Sheraton or the Carlton or luxury resorts such as Bintin Island in Indonesia and the Royal Cliff Beach Resort in Pattaya, Thailand. I usually travel business class, which is noted, of course, for its extra leg room! I often joke to the airline staff: 'Perhaps I should sub-lease my leg room? Look, I could get another family over here in front of me!'

My wife Elaine often travels with me (in her own seat I hasten to add), so we are able to mix business with pleasure and enjoy some sightseeing as well. To me, being a professional speaker is not so much a job as a passion. I never fail to find it exciting and at the age of

I can't believe life is so good and so full of promise for the future.

Some people have told me I'm lucky I got run over by a train and lost my legs because they say adversity makes you a better person. They reckon such a challenge in your life makes you dig down deep inside and that it brings out the best in you. My answer to that is: why do we wait? Why do people waste their lives sitting around waiting for something to happen — waiting to get run over by a train — before they get out there and do something about it? Having said that, my accident has shaped my character and life in many ways and it certainly helps me to get my inspirational message across.

During my presentations I like to take people on an emotional roller-coaster ride by first explaining how I lost my legs and then how I've faced the challenges of life without them.

Although it was more than 30 years ago, I still remember the day of my accident like it was yesterday. It was the winter of 1967 and I was nine years old. I'd gone with a friend and his father one Saturday morning to help bag coal from a couple of wagons at the Te Maunga railway yard on the outskirts of Tauranga. My friend Gary's dad belonged to the local branch of the Lions Club that raised funds for community projects. The coal had been donated to the Lions Club so they could bag it up and sell it in aid of different charities. It was Queen's Birthday weekend and about 20 volunteers turned up to help unload the wagons. Gary and I were given the task of delivering empty sacks from the back of a truck to the wagons that were sitting on a track in the middle of the railway yard. The men would then shovel the coal into the sacks and carry them back to the truck. To get to and from the coal wagons we had to walk around another train. We could either go the long way round in front of the engine or take a short cut around the back of the wagons, the last of which was a 40-tonne flat-deck carrying a big bulldozer. Naturally, we opted for the short cut and it was as we were crossing the line behind the flat-deck that the train suddenly shunted backwards for no apparent reason, hitting me on my left shoulder and dragging me under. Dual sets of wheels ran over both my legs, nearly severing them, and the miracle was that I survived the shock and horrendous loss of blood. But survive I did, although my badly mangled legs had to be amputated above the knee.

I spent the next seven months in and out of Tauranga Hospital. While my family and friends struggled to cope with the shock of my accident, the people of Tauranga rallied around with great generosity, support and spirit.

I was fitted with my first artificial legs, which were very basic aluminium and steel jobs, and finally went back to school — in a wheelchair. Thanks to the teachers there I fitted well into school life. My new legs weren't totally adequate and I spent a lot of time with them off, in my chair or shuffling on my bum — even climbing trees. I also got about on trolleys and a bike and joined in with my mates among the neighbourhood kids. My sister Sue also let me ride her horse, but anything more than a trot was too much to handle.

I couldn't race off with the other kids but when I was left behind I wasn't idle. I developed my artistic side, drawing boyish things on a big pad: racing cars, dragsters and planes. With Dad, I put together models of planes and boats.

I was determined to do the things I did before the accident, and my family and friends were keen for me to have a normal life too. I was an outgoing, boisterous kid — perhaps a bit of a handful at times — and no one was going to hide me away. I wanted to be independent, not mollycoddled.

As a child I hated water and couldn't swim, but that didn't stop Dave Franklin and Allan Guthrie, Tauranga swimming coaches and friends of my parents, deciding swimming would be excellent physiotherapy for me. At my first lesson, they didn't ask me to get in the pool; I was unceremoniously thrown in. I sank to the bottom; my coaches fished me out with a net used for skimming leaves from the pool. It wasn't an auspicious start, but my coaches didn't give up and nor did I. In time I learnt to float, then learnt to swim. I also learnt an important lesson about coping with my 'disability': if I wanted to do something, I couldn't spend time wondering if I could do it — I had to get out there and just do it.

Five months after my first lesson, I swam a mile, 52 lengths of the pool, without stopping. I joined the swim club and practised continually, becoming a strong swimmer. With some compensation money received from the Railways, my parents built a backyard pool. Once it was completed, I was in it every day, doing lengths. My ability at swimming let me set some goals for myself, entering races and enjoying competition. I never spent much time sitting around at home. Mum and Dad always encouraged me to get out and participate. Through my involvement with the Crippled Children's Society I realised I wasn't the only person with challenges, and I also discovered there were people who would help, if you asked.

Trips to Baypark Raceway got me interested in racing, and soon I was behind the wheel of a go-kart. This was an activity that I was able to do together with my father. I also loved to spend time with my grandad, going fishing and chatting about boats and cars.

At intermediate and high school, I was a little unruly at times (well, perhaps, lots of times), and my teachers didn't regard me as the prime candidate for academic success. My swim coach, Dave Franklin, suggested I get involved in surf lifesaving, and thus began a new adventure for me. I joined the Omanu Pacific Surf Club as a surf lifeguard, and thoroughly enjoyed the involvement. I was able to save 33 lives and in recognition gained a certificate from the World Lifesaving Federation. That was important to me, as I was being honoured for my achievement as a lifeguard, regardless of the fact that I didn't have any legs.

Surf lifesaving taught me about commitment to something and the benefits of training and practice, as well as leadership and teamwork skills. I also enjoyed the friendship and comradeship, and the joy of competing.

About the same time that I got into surf lifesaving I became involved with the disabled sports movement, learning to throw the discus, shot put and javelin, and racing in wheelchairs, along with swimming. It gave me the chance to compete in sports like other teenage guys, and before long I was representing New Zealand. In 1975, with great excitement, I embarked on my first overseas trip as a member of the team chosen for the disabled games in Oita, Japan. I won a silver and two golds there. I felt it was a phenomenal achievement for me, and it proved to me that you should dream; and, if you tried hard enough, you could achieve that dream.

I went on to represent New Zealand five times at different World, Paralympic and FESPIC (Far Eastern and South Pacific Games for the Handicapped) games, winning 35 medals during my athletics career, visiting several countries, making many friends and having numerous adventures with my fellow competitors. I stopped competing in athletics when in my late twenties as other commitments took over: a business, a young family and motor sports.

I was determined that I wasn't going to be any different from any of my mates. I had learned to drive and had my own car, which had been adapted to suit me, and this gave me great independence (sometimes to my parents' horror) and I did all the things young men my age did. I had a girlfriend, I went to parties, I worked on and hooned around in my car. I became really interested in racing, but before I could get involved properly, I landed my first job. I had left school at 16, never the great scholar, but with a wealth of experience and travel under my belt. I became a ticket writer at Woolworths, writing prices on cards, and soon moved on to a rival supermarket, New World. At 17 I had my own office, a regular wage, and grew in confidence as I felt I was treated like an equal member of staff. Before long, I had moved into signwriting, not an easy transition as most signwriting firms rebuffed my approaches, citing my inability to climb a ladder or drive a truck. I first worked for the Tauranga Museum, where I learnt the skills to work professionally as a signwriter. Also at the museum was Jim Muir, who was doing screenprinting. Before long, we had teamed up and started our own signwriting and screenprinting business. During this time I met Jim's neighbour, Elaine, the girl I would later marry. I eventually bought Jim out and carried on the business by myself, achieving my dream of owning my own business by the time I was 30 with two years to spare.

Despite the misgivings of some observers, my relationship with Elaine blossomed, and we started living together. Elaine had a daughter, Nikki, from a previous marriage, and on 1 March 1979, I became a father for the first time, to Danielle. Managing a baby tested all my coping powers, I must admit.

Elaine and I got married on 27 October 1979, just four days after my twenty-first birthday. By then we had moved to our home in Welcome Bay near Tauranga. Three years later, Lucas was born. As children do, they completely accepted my legless state and we enjoyed ourselves just as any family would. Over the years there were numerous articles in the local newspaper about me and my achievements, so my children sometimes suffered a lack of privacy from having a 'famous' father, but otherwise nothing has interfered with them becoming well-rounded adults who have achieved their own goals.

I went back to go-kart racing, becoming good enough to compete at events around the North Island. I then got interested in speedway and bought a midget car. Ever competitive and determined, I won championships at Baypark, Western Springs and Meremere. Later I also tried the Pre-65 class, which is slower and less stressful. It is expensive and not without its dangers (and I've had the odd spill) but I love motor racing. I don't care whether I win or lose, it is just being out there competing that makes me happy. And if it has an engine on it, point me at it — I want to give it a try — sidecar racing, jetskis, off-road biking, you name it.

In 1986 I found a new challenge — the martial art of tae kwon do.

Nikki was taking lessons and her tutor suggested I follow suit. After three years of training I obtained my first-degree black belt, and then taught the sport. In 1990 I gained my second-degree black belt.

Always in search of a fresh adventure, I created aviation history in March 1998 by being the first person with a disability to learn to fly solo. I'm still keen on flying and aim to keep my hours up by regular flights, but it is an expensive hobby. I also took to the air in another way, during an exhilarating tandem parachute dive.

I loved every minute of my time as a signwriter and businessman. I still get a kick out of seeing so many of my signs on display all over Tauranga. They were fun times, but after 12 years new opportunities presented themselves and I began setting new goals. After a few speaking engagements resulted in a warm reception from listeners, a new career as a professional speaker took shape.

I may not have quite achieved my dream of becoming the best inspirational speaker in the world yet but I'm well on the way and it is a goal I'm working hard at. In the past 12 months I've had more than 150 speaking engagements, the biggest of which was in front of 11,000 people at the Asia and Pacific Life Insurers' Conference in Singapore earlier this year. Last year I addressed 8000 delegates at the Million Dollar Round Table Conference in Toronto. I was very proud of that engagement because at that stage I'd only been in the business just over four years and I know of speakers who've been around 15 years or more who would give their eye teeth to talk to such a prestigious group.

Despite Elaine's initial fears when I sold my signwriting business to venture into the unknown world of professional speaking, she's now the first to admit that as a result of that gamble everything in our lives has improved tremendously:

> *'I must confess I was anxious when Tony told me he wanted to become an inspirational speaker. And certainly the first year was hard financially because he was new to the circuit and not so*

well known. But he was determined to achieve his goal and since then things have just snowballed to the stage where everything about our lives is bigger and better. I guess he's applied all the principles to his own life that he talks about in his presentations. He's always had dreams and set goals and he's always had the courage and determination to turn them into reality. Sure it was a risk financially but if you don't try you'll never know what you can or can't achieve and you could end up being haunted for the rest of your life by lost opportunities.

'When Tony had the signwriting business I used to help him with the office work and now it is my job to handle all his bookings, accounts and travel arrangements. I love it because I can work from home and I also go along with him on overseas trips sometimes and I really enjoy that. We've been to some wonderful places and we usually manage to fit in a bit of sightseeing around his speaking engagements. His change of career came at a good time in our lives because our three children have grown up now so we can come and go without having to worry about them. When Tony used to trip around the world with his sport I wasn't able to travel with him because we had young children and we couldn't afford for both of us to go. And later I had a job as a head chef, which meant I couldn't just take time off whenever I wanted — whereas Tony's work allowed him time to compete overseas. Now we seem to be making up for lost time and in the past three or four years we've had countless trips across the Tasman together as well as to the States, Fiji, Vanuatu and Singapore.

'When I do go along with him I usually get the job of selling his books, CD and video after his presentation and I really enjoy meeting all the people and listening to their feedback. It makes me feel very proud of Tony and all he's achieved.'

When I'm not working or playing with my grandchildren or putting the finishing touches to the house (my wife reckons I'll make a great tiler if ever I tire of being a speaker) I still manage to find time for a few hobbies. I love rally driving whenever I have the opportunity and I race my sprint car at Mt Maunganui's Baypark Speedway every weekend throughout summer when I'm home. I still like to get behind the controls of a single-engine aircraft whenever I get the time and I'm currently learning to fly a remote-controlled helicopter. I've just gained my scuba diver's certificate so now I'm looking forward to exploring some of the underwater wonders both in New Zealand and overseas.

Unfortunately, I don't have much time to devote to tae kwon do these days but I do make the effort, when I'm home, to play wheelchair basketball once a week and in summertime my five-year-old grandson Houston loves to go out on the harbour with me on my jetski.

I lost my legs 35 years ago and although I can still remember the accident and the ensuing months vividly, I certainly haven't wasted my life worrying about what might have been had I not gone to the railway yard with Gary and his dad that day. People tell me I'm lucky — I've got a loving wife, a healthy family, a great job and I've been successful in many aspects of my life. But I can't agree with them. Luck is winning the lottery. I'm fortunate — fortunate that I have been able to get out and do so many things in my life, that my kids are well and happy and that I met Elaine.

But I've also worked hard to achieve things in my life, and I've learnt a few things along the way. So before I tell you any more about my adventures in Africa I'd like to share some thoughts with you on the importance of setting goals, making the right choices, taking risks and dreaming dreams.

2 making a difference

It's great to be able to make a difference to people's lives.

Seeking inspiration and inspiring others

I have often said that I'm not a motivational speaker; I aim to be an inspirational speaker. I tell a story and hope listeners will be inspired enough by it to make a change or make a difference in their lives. I believe that we can change and we can do anything we want. If just one person can read one of my books or watch my video or go away from my presentation feeling inspired enough to make positive changes to their life then I'll have done my job. Judging from the great feedback I receive, people do find my message inspiring, which is great because it comes from the heart.

In fact sometimes it seems I can inspire people too much! I had one employer ring me from Australia after I'd addressed a conference. He said he'd really enjoyed my talk and his staff had thought it fantastic too. Only trouble was, three of them had been so inspired they'd all tendered their resignation the next day! But instead of being displeased their boss said he really wanted to thank me because they were all people who'd been thinking about doing other things for some time. He said I'd shown them how to overcome the fear

You can do anything you want to. You just have to want to do it badly enough.

factor and go out and accept the challenges they were looking for but until then had been too afraid to do anything about. He said he admired their courage and sincerely hoped they would succeed in their new ventures. I guess he realised that if those staff members were no longer happy working for him then he wasn't getting their full potential from them. Hopefully, his understanding attitude and encouragement would in itself be an inspiration, to all his employees.

Inspiration's a bit like that: it can have a spin-off effect. It often only takes one member of a group or family to achieve a goal for all the other members to want to follow suit. Your enthusiasm for life can fire up someone else and they can pass it on down the line.

You don't have to be successful at everything you do, but at least have the courage to set yourself goals and then do your best to achieve them. That's all you can ask of yourself: that you do your best. How do we know what our capabilities are unless we give something our best shot? That is certainly what I have always tried to do. Whatever I set out to achieve I put in 100 per cent effort. I know no other way. I don't always succeed, but at least I know I couldn't have tried any harder. Like when I'm motor racing, for example. I can't win all the time, although of course I'd like to! But when I get behind the wheel of my car and strap my helmet on and fire up the engine the adrenalin starts to flow and I go out there to do the very best that I can. I love every minute of it, despite all the trials and tribulations — and believe me, there are plenty of those in motor racing! There's so much to think about and be aware of as you whizz around the track but for me it is all a tremendous buzz. Because I'm trying as hard as I can it doesn't matter what position I finish in: first, third or last. When I drive into the pits at the end of the race I feel like a winner because I've given it my best shot and had a damn good time to boot. Even if I come

> *Inspiration often has a spin-off effect. Your enthusiasm can fire up someone else and they in turn inspire others.*

second to last, hey — there's still one other car behind me and I've beaten it! If someone sees me out there having fun and is encouraged and inspired to give motor racing a go themselves, then that's a bonus.

It is great to be able to make a difference to people's lives. I especially like talking to schoolchildren, and Elaine and I love the letters we receive from them afterwards. When I'm talking to schools I usually throw in lots of physical stuff like tae kwon do moves, flip-overs, press-ups and hand stands and I tell them all about my sporting interests. I tell them how proud I was to represent my country at five World Games and what it is like to stand on the dais when you've won a gold medal and hear your national anthem being played over the loud speaker. I tell them about the medals I've won and I give them some idea of the amount of training and dedication that's needed to be a successful athlete. I try to encourage them to think about what it is they want out of life and to understand the importance of having ambitions and aspirations. New Zealand is a very sporting nation and there are so many 'home-grown' heroes the young kids of today can identify with, whether they be All Blacks, Tall Blacks, Black Caps, Black Sox or Silver Ferns.

You don't have to succeed at everything, but at least have the courage to set yourself goals and then do your best to achieve them.

My new career has meant I am in contact with more people than ever before, and I feel I have the opportunity to help people, in some small way, make changes in their lives. As Elaine says:

> 'One of the great things about what he does now, which we know from all the correspondence we get, is that he's making a difference to people's lives. I remember in particular a young woman telling me once that she'd been born with a face 'only a mother could love' and that she'd been brought up 'the hard way' and made some terrible mistakes in her life. But she said that

through reading Tony's first book, Race You to the Top, *she'd been able to turn her life around. I thought that was terrific.'*

Some of my sources of inspiration

Along with thousands of other New Zealand schoolboys, my heroes when I was young were the country's most prominent sports stars. Back then Colin (Pinetree) Meads and Kel Tremain were two of the biggest All Black stars, and I remember the thrill of having them both visit me in Tauranga Hospital not long after my accident. Colin brought me a six-panelled football that had been signed by the 1959 Lions and All Black teams and I still have it proudly displayed in my office.

You can imagine what it did for my morale to have two of my childhood heroes take the time to come and see me. I've still got the photo that appeared in the local paper of Colin handing me the ball. I've met the All Black legend a number of times in recent years, and he still remembers visiting me in hospital. Those were the days before sport turned professional, of course. These days rugby players behave and expect to be treated (and paid) like film stars, but when Colin Meads was an All Black he worked on his King Country farm on the Friday, played a test match on the Saturday, club rugby on the Sunday and was back on the farm the next day. To me he's one of the true icons of New Zealand sport, but as he said, before giving the following comments, he still finds all the attention a little embarrassing at times.

Colin Meads was a giant of the rugby world who was a hero to thousands of New Zealand schoolboys. His visit gave me an incredible boost.

'I still remember going to see Tony in hospital seven or eight days after he'd had his accident. I was in Tauranga to play for either King Country or Maniapoto at the time, I'm not sure which, and an old chap who was a great rugby man there took me along to *see him. I think he took Kel Tremain to see him a week or so later when Hawke's Bay were playing in Tauranga. I can remember giving Tony the autographed ball and, like him, I've still got the newspaper cutting showing me handing it to him. The six-panelled rugby ball was an experimental one and it was only used in New Zealand for about a year in 1959, but I always liked it because it gave you a better grip than a four-panel ball. Anyway, Tony was obviously still in shock after losing his legs and I remember he was a very quiet kid, but very polite. I used to get quite a thrill out of being able to do things like that; to visit people in hospital and feel that I'd been able to cheer them up a bit. I think the All Blacks still do that sort of thing today, which is great. Then I met up with Tony again some years ago when I was invited to open the Eve Rimmer Games in Whakatane. He made himself known and the next day I went to watch him play basketball. I remember thinking, 'You cruel buggers,' because they were really rough, ramming into each other and tipping one another out of their chairs. Since then our paths have crossed several times and it has been great to see the bubbly person he's become, so full of life. He's a very inspirational guy and one who has overcome tremendous handicaps; he just brushes it off like it is not there. It doesn't worry him. And you don't help Tony. He's got an 'I can do it my bloody self' sort of attitude because he's that sort of guy.'*

These days Colin and his wife Verna have a sheep and beef farm in Te Kuiti, just a mile up the road from the family property where he grew up and where one of his sons now lives. Not that he gets to spend much time there. He does a lot of promotional work for the Australian-based tanalised timber company, Koppers Arch, and he also gets invited to speak at a lot of functions because of his rugby connections. The week he spoke to me for this book he had flown down to Wellington on a

Friday for a Rugby Foundation charity function at which he was guest speaker. He flew back on the Saturday to watch his 15-year-old grandson Clinton competing in school rowing championships and then two days later he and Verna were off back to Wellington for a Parliamentary luncheon in honour of Sir Edmund Hillary. Then it was up to Auckland for a tribute dinner for former Olympic runner John Walker. At last year's inaugural tribute dinner it was Colin who was the guest of honour.

People like Colin Meads and Sir Edmund Hillary represent the kind of 'living legends' who achieved things outside of their normal working lives, in the days before professional sport, at least in this country. We still have our sporting greats, but they don't have to do a 'proper' job during the week to put food on the table, attend training sessions after work at night and then be expected to play for nothing at the weekend. Those days have long gone.

If I were to choose the person who most inspired me as a youngster I would have to say Sir Douglas Bader. For those too young to remember, Englishman Douglas Bader became a legend in his lifetime for his courage and determination, especially during the Second World War, when he earned medals for bravery for his flying exploits despite being, like me, a double amputee. Bader lost his legs at the age of 21, when he crashed his RAF Bristol Bulldog fighter while attempting to perform aerobatics. As with my accident, his legs were so badly mangled they had to be amputated. He wasn't expected to survive. Within a couple of years, however, he was walking again, albeit on artificial legs, and he also had a car modified so that he could resume driving. It took him a little bit longer to persuade the RAF to let him back at the controls of a plane, but on 27 November 1939, eight years after his crash, he flew solo again at the controls of an Avro Tudor K-3242. After that there was no stopping him and he was awarded the Distinguished Flying Cross and the Distinguished Service Order for gallantry and leadership of the highest order during the Battle of

Britain. In 1941 Bader was captured by the Germans after a mid-air collision with a Messerschmitt Me-109 and he spent the rest of the war in captivity, some of it at the infamous Colditz prison, where, despite having no legs, he tried several times to escape. In 1976 he was knighted for his services to amputees, 'so many of whom he had helped and inspired by his example and character'. But it wasn't just amputees he inspired. Through his flying exploits he'd become a real-life hero to men and boys all over the world, so you can imagine how I felt when, at the age of 10, I got to meet him in the flesh!

After the war Douglas Bader became worldwide marketing manager for the Shell Oil Company and it just so happened that my father worked for Shell in Tauranga as a tanker driver. Bader was visiting New Zealand on business and my father's boss and colleagues got together the money to fly Dad and me up to Auckland to meet him. It was only about a year after I'd lost my legs and it was a truly amazing experience for me. We were only supposed to spend 10 or 20 minutes with him in his hotel room but an hour and a half later we were still talking. I can still remember him vividly. He was wearing an old tweed suit and carried a walking stick and he spoke with a very English accent. One of his aides said to him, 'Mr Bader, we've got to go now,' and he turned around and looked at me and said, 'I'm not leaving this young man just yet.' I'll never forget that.

It only takes one person to make a difference in your life. Meeting Douglas Bader inspired me to fight for what I think is right and to believe in my own abilities.

Douglas Bader had such a charismatic air about him, and I'm sure the things he told me that day inspired me to go out and fight for what I wanted in life. He told me stories about the war and why he'd carried on flying after his accident. He said flying was part of his life and he believed the fact that he'd lost his legs didn't make any difference to the way he could fly an aeroplane. He also told me about how he'd had to battle bureaucracy to be allowed back in the air, and I think what he told me that day has subconsciously stayed with me and helped get me where I am today. My meeting with him taught me not to take no for an answer and to fight for what I think is right and to believe in my own abilities.

It only takes one person to make a difference in your life, and to have met Douglas Bader at that stage of my life was probably the best thing that could have happened to me.

Heroes, however, are not just phenomena of the twentieth or twenty-first centuries. If you go back through history you find hundreds of people who've set themselves goals and pursued their dreams and achieved results in all kinds of fields: Thomas Edison, Florence Nightingale, George Washington, Leonardo da Vinci. They all had several things in common. They were dreamers. They were goal setters. They were passionate. They knew what they wanted and they had the desire to succeed.

It is not just the famous achievers who make an impression on me, though. I'm not a great reader or television viewer and so I tend to be more inspired by the people and things I see in real life. For instance, I couldn't help but be inspired by some of the people I met in tribal villages during my trip to Africa. They had so little in the way of modern-day possessions and their life expectancy was so short and yet they seemed incredibly happy and contented with their lives. They didn't seem burdened with what I call 'excess baggage', all those negative feelings of greed, envy or jealousy or the desire to 'keep up with the Joneses'.

In the Western world today everybody wants everything whether they can afford it or not. They just flash their plastic cards and book things up regardless of the cost. We see the commercials on television and think, 'Oh … I must have that.' If we don't get what we want then we're consumed with frustration, anguish and envy. But the Masai people have never had any of the luxury items that so many of us take for granted. They don't have wall-to-wall carpet, television, DVDs, computers, refrigerators, microwaves or *en suite* facilities. Many don't even have flush toilets and they certainly don't have malls and megastores out on the steppes or the Serengeti. So they don't know what they're missing. I think that's why they're so happy. Their wants, needs and expectations are very simple and indeed they probably consider themselves rich and privileged compared with other tribes in Africa. I don't believe money and possessions necessarily make you any happier; on the other hand, if you're lucky enough to live in a land full of opportunities, as many of us do, then in my opinion it is a crime to let those opportunities pass you by.

The Masai people I met didn't appear burdened with greed, envy or jealousy.

One of the earliest influences on my life was my maternal grandfather, Frank Sherman, who died in 1997 at the age of 93. He was a jack of all trades and master of none but to me he was just the greatest. When I had my accident he and Nana were living at Whenuapai, near Auckland, on the flight path to the Whenuapai Air Base, and I think that's where my life-long passion for aviation really began. He and I would sit on the roof of his house for hours and hours watching the planes come and go. They flew so low over us that you could just about reach up and touch their wheels, or so it seemed when I was a kid. It was around that time that I started collecting and flying model aircraft, a hobby I still enjoy.

Later my grandparents moved to Omokoroa on the outskirts of Tauranga, and Wednesday was always my favourite day of the week because that's the day they'd come into town to do their shopping and then have dinner with us. I'd sit beside my grandad and listen to him talk for hours about electricity and boats or cars and engines and how to make things work. He taught me so many interesting things and we had such a lot of fun together. He had a wonderfully dry sense of humour, but I guess he was also a bit of an eccentric and I must admit he did some strange things sometimes. Like the time he painted his vinyl lounge suite because he didn't like the colour. Unfortunately, when he and Nana sat on it the vinyl sweated and all the paint cracked and stuck to their clothes! Another time he made a magnificent full-sized billiards table down in the basement only to find he couldn't get it through the door and upstairs into the house. Not a problem to dear old Grandad. He simply shifted the table outside and built another room right around it.

> *Grandad was a talented, inventive, eccentric man and a great storyteller. I greatly admired how he coped with a very bad stutter.*

I suppose the thing I admired most about him, though, was the way he coped with the fact that he had a very bad stutter. It wasn't the sort of speech impediment where he repeated the same letter over and over again; his problem was he sometimes just couldn't get any sound out at all. I obviously don't take after him in that respect! It must have been a real challenge in his life and his mates use to tease and mimic him, but it never seemed to worry him too much. I learnt as a young boy, though, to never try to help him when he was struggling to say a word. Even if I could tell what it was he was trying to say I knew to just sit there patiently and wait for him to get it out.

Besides being a wonderful storyteller Grandad was also a bit of an inventor and long before remote controls came on the market he actually made himself a gadget that did a similar sort of job. He had a dog called Rexy, who used to howl every time the advertisements came on television. (I'm sure many of us can identify with Rexy on that score!) Anyway, there was no way he could cure the dog of this annoying habit and so he rigged up a small bracket with string attached to it so that he could sit in his armchair and just pull the string to turn the volume down whenever the commercials came on. Likewise, once the ads were over he could turn the volume back up again and Rexy was none the wiser.

I believe these days we're missing out on some wonderful stories and talents that older people could pass on to us because we either don't ask them or we don't take the time to listen. Our grandparents have so many great anecdotes and trade secrets from the past that I'm sure they'd love to share. They could teach the kids of today so much if they would care to listen. If you have an elderly relative or neighbour, make an effort to find out their life story; you might well be amazed at the things they have achieved. Remember, we all have stories in our lives that are just waiting to be passed on.

We all have stories ready to be passed on. Make an effort to hear others' stories.

People like Grandad, Sir Douglas Bader and Colin Meads were my childhood heroes, but I found plenty of others who inspired me once I began competing in international sporting events. It was during this period of my life, in my late teens and early twenties, that I had so many unforgettable experiences, such as seeing Olympic blind runners finishing the 100 metres event just fractions of a second slower than the world able-bodied 100 metres' record. There were Olympic high jumpers too, who, with one only one leg, jumped just centimetres less than the world able-bodied high-jump record.

I know from experience that these 'disabled' athletes train just as hard as able-bodied athletes and that the competition is just as tough. But, alas, all too often their glory and their triumphs go unappreciated and unacknowledged in their own country.

I've mentioned a few of the people who really inspired me as a youngster but there is another person, who though not well known, had a great effect on my life a few years later. Fay Goodall, a very dear friend, sadly died a year ago. She taught me so much about myself and my attitude to life. Fay and her husband John both had cerebral palsy. They lived not far from Tauranga, in Te Puke, the 'kiwifruit capital of the world'. Elaine and I first met them early on in our married life when our kids were still very young. We went to picturesque Lake

Okataina, near Rotorua, one weekend with a group of 'disabled' people. About six or seven families, including Fay and John, stayed together at Okataina Lodge. We arrived on the Friday evening and it was a black, wet night. Weatherwise it didn't look as if the weekend was going to be very good at all. We put the kids to bed in the bunkhouse and then all the adults gathered in a little lounge in front of a big open fire. We sat around talking for a while and then we began to play games. Fay and I were playing Connect Four. It is a bit like noughts and crosses only you drop counters into a little frame and have to form a line of four. Now although John's speech was a little slurred as a result of his palsy, his mobility was quite good, but Fay was fairly badly incapacitated. Her body was twisted like so many who suffer from the condition and it was difficult to understand what she was saying unless you really took the time to listen to her. She couldn't dress herself or do any of the other daily chores most of us take for granted and she could only get around very slowly with John holding onto her arm. Despite all the difficulties they faced in life, they were a really lovely couple and you never heard them complain.

On this particular Friday night Fay was very slowly picking up her counters, one at a time, and dropping them into the Connect Four frame, her hand shaking with the effort it took to lift them off the table. I was feeling a real smart young fellow and as she slowly let go of her counter, I'd be holding mine over the edge of the frame ready to drop it in too. I'd keep urging her on, saying, 'Come on, Fay, you can do it, you can do it.' Each time, as she slowly dropped her counter in and before it had even hit the bottom, I'd have dropped mine in as well. But despite my speed and enthusiasm, at the end of the session Fay had won four out of five

> *To see the difficulties other people have in their lives and observe how they overcome them is both humbling and inspirational. I learnt a lot from the way Fay Goodall coped with the challenges in her life.*

games, which rather took me down a peg or two because I'm a very competitive person and I'd been so full of confidence.

We spent the rest of the weekend going for bush walks, looking for wallabies and glow-worms, playing cricket and generally having a lot of fun. The Sunday was a reasonably clear day and so we took Fay and John out in our boat and they enjoyed being with us and the kids. We went home on the Sunday evening and a couple of days later we got a letter from Fay. It had been typed and was beautifully composed. She said what a wonderful time she'd had at Okataina and as she mentioned the different things we'd done it was like painting a picture in our minds so that we could almost smell the pine trees and see the glow-worms again. At the bottom of the letter she had written: 'PS. I enjoyed beating Tony at Connect Four!'

That night I rang John and asked him to thank Fay for her letter. I said how much we'd appreciated it and that in fact the kids had taken it to school for 'show and tell' time. In his slurred speech John proudly informed me that it had taken Fay four and a half hours to type that letter. He said she'd done it by hitting the keys with a pencil that she held in her mouth. It was at that moment I realised how frustrating it must be for such an intelligent mind to be trapped in a body that won't work. Most of us talk about the frustrations we face in our lives today but nothing can compare to the challenges that Fay went through every day of her life. That night at Okataina I was being such a smart aleck, thinking I was so clever, when all the time she had me really sorted out.

The more I've thought about that in the intervening years the more I've come to understand what life must have been like for Fay and I realise how much she taught me. We all make a difference in someone's life and she certainly made a difference in mine that night.

Some ways to inspire and be inspired

I really do believe that we all have it in us to inspire someone else. You don't have to lead an action-packed life or be an astute businessperson or a great academic. It is possible to inspire someone just by a look or a word given at the right time. A sympathetic shoulder to cry on could be all somebody needs to give them the confidence to make a change in their life. You might think you lead a very quiet, uneventful, humdrum life but to those whose lives are always frenetic and disorganised that can be very inspiring. Or the fact that you stand up for something you believe in or go out and get a job or enrol for a night-school course could inspire someone you barely know to follow your example. How many times have you admired a quality in someone else and thought to yourself: 'I must try and be more like him or her'?

There are other ways of being inspired as well. Just by reading about someone's achievement in a newspaper you can think: 'Well, if they can do it why shouldn't I give it a go?' Everyone has different dreams and goals and they're not all to do with fame or glory or medals or money. More often than not, satisfaction or pride in your achievement is the best reward. As the nineteenth-century American poet Ralph Waldo Emerson once noted, 'The reward of a thing well done is to have done it.' It is as simple as that. Some people dream of paddling a kayak around New Zealand or sailing single-handed across the Pacific. Others might want to swim Cook Strait or across Lake Taupo or run in a marathon. Or just stay home and be the best mum or dad they can be. It doesn't matter how mundane your goal might seem to others, if it is important to you, then go for it. Remember, you're never too old to make dreams come true.

We can all inspire others, sometimes with just a look or a word given at the right time.

I read recently about a Bay of Plenty man, Tom Bayliss, who'd been a teacher all his life and often, while in the classroom, he'd dreamt of going walkabout, as the Australian Aborigines call it, with just a pack on his back. So, in his sixties, a year or two after he retired, that's exactly what he did. Every summer for three years Tom set off from his home in Whakatane to walk around the coastline of the North Island. He'd get as far as he could in eight to 10 weeks and then return to his home town to resume his part-time duties as a children's music-school teacher as well as his role as conductor of the local community orchestra. Then the following summer he'd resume his walk where he'd left off the previous year, taking with him only a small tent, a change of clothes and a small amount of food. This year he finished the last leg of the walk and came home triumphant. He'd achieved his goal and the experience was everything he'd dreamt it would be and more. He'd learnt so much about his country, its people and, most importantly, about himself and his capabilities. Now he's being kept busy sharing those experiences with others as guest speaker for various local clubs. After all that walking, he says he has never felt fitter in his life.

Everyone should have dreams. I never have trouble going to sleep because every night when I go to bed I dream about all the things I want to do with my life and that's what helps me to nod off. I'm able to take my mind and put it somewhere where I want to be or doing something that I want to do and I can picture it in my mind. I think visualisation is a great part of goal setting. For example, if I'm motor racing the next day I can go to bed the night before and close my eyes and see myself out there on the track — usually giving the victory sign as I take the chequered flag!

Regardless of how mundane your goal might seem to others, if it is important to you, then go for it.

At the moment I'm learning how to fly a remote-controlled helicopter and so every night after I've been playing with the simulator on the computer I go to sleep dreaming about flying my helicopter. Of course, some people only dream and don't try turning their dreams into reality but that's their choice. Hopefully, some may find the courage to go that extra step.

Some years ago there was story on television about a very personable elderly Maori man from Rotorua called Roger Kusabs. In his late eighties, Roger found himself crippled with painful arthritis and felt his life really wasn't worth living any more. Then his doctor put him on an all fruit and vegetable diet and told him to take up jogging. The old man told the doctor not to be so stupid, pointing out that he was in so much pain that he couldn't even walk to the gate and back. So the doctor told him to just walk as far as he could each day and to stick to the diet and see if his health improved.

Well, within a year Roger was jogging around Arawa Racecourse every morning before breakfast and feeling half his age. Given this new lease of life he then looked for something interesting to occupy his time and mind, and after doing some market research, he decided there were no decent popguns in the local toyshops. So he designed a wooden re-loadable popgun and began mass-producing it out of off-cuts he collected from the nearby Waipa Sawmill. He cut the bits of wood into fun shapes — triangles, circles and the like — and got his grandchildren to help dunk them in buckets of brightly coloured non-toxic dye. It was a simple but ingenious design, and to Roger's delight it sold like hot cakes all over New Zealand. After being featured on television he was recognised as 'the popgun man' wherever he went and he revelled in his new-found fame and fortune. For several years into his nineties the enterprising old fellow could afford to buy himself a new car every year and have an annual trip to Australia. He even carted a carton of popguns over to Sydney with him, and the toys were snapped up there too. In fact such was the demand that had he been younger he'd have probably set up a factory and gone into mass production, exporting them all over the world. He could have become a millionaire, but he was happy just to have been able to turn his life around and get some excitement and fulfilment out of his last few years. Only a year or two earlier he'd thought his life wasn't worth living any more.

When he died in 1999 at the age of 100, his son Andrew was besieged with letters from people he'd never heard of before wanting to share 'popgun stories' with him. He said he hadn't realised until then just how many lives his much-loved father had touched through his enthusiasm for life and his simple invention.

It is never too late to change your life around, to have a good idea and run with it, to have a dream and turn it into reality.

Roger's story really appealed to me as an example of how challenges can be met and overcome, and I know there are thousands of other inspirational stories like that just waiting to be told. Everyone has a cross to bear in life, be it a physical or mental challenge, the indignities of old age, financial stress or relationship problems. But life is still the most precious commodity there is no matter how hard the going gets. Don't ever give up on it. There's nearly always a solution to every problem, although some people have a bigger struggle than others to find it.

I recently read of a Japanese man who celebrated his ninety-ninth birthday by skiing down the highest mountain in western Europe, Mont Blanc in the French Alps. Not surprisingly, officials believed him to be the oldest person to make the descent. What's more, he was accompanied by his 70-year-old son and 37-year-old grandson. He'd long been an accomplished mountaineer and skier, but to undertake such a feat at his age was quite remarkable. The first part of the descent was so steep it had to be made on foot and the old man had to trudge through the snow with his skis on his back.

There are thousands of senior citizens all around the world fulfilling life-long dreams by doing something adventurous like skiing, skydiving or bungy jumping. However, not all goals have to be the adrenalin-pumping variety. Some people write books in their retirement, or take up a new hobby such as fishing or playing bridge.

One 90-year-old Whakatane woman had always wanted to play a musical instrument and, at the age of 88, she began learning to play the flute. Do you know how much puff it takes to play one of those things? But that didn't deter Juliette Stonyer, or the fact that she couldn't read music and that her fingers were deformed by arthritis. Her happy, youthful and positive attitude gave her the confidence to give it a go and by all accounts she is doing really well. In fact the last I heard she was enjoying making music so much that she'd set herself another goal. She hopes one day to be good enough to play in the local community orchestra, and her teacher says she has the determination and the ability to achieve that goal. Good for her!

Learning to swim was the catalyst that made me realise I could still be one of life's achievers even though I no longer had legs. Once I'd learnt to swim well, I couldn't wait to tackle other challenges. I no longer dwelt on all the things I couldn't do with my mates; instead, I went out looking for activities I could participate in. This led to surf lifesaving and involvement in the disabled sports movement, which opened up whole new worlds for me. Since then I've tried my hand at all kinds of sports, and hopefully I'll still be pushing boundaries in my old age.

No matter how old or how young you are, there's absolutely no excuse for anyone to be bored. If you're not into sport and the great outdoors then look at all the fun you can have in the comfort of your own home with PlayStations, radio, television, videos, CDs, DVDs and the like. There's no need to be lonely, either, thanks to the advent of email and text messaging. The Internet can bring the whole world into your lounge and it is a great learning tool for adults as well as children. Leading a somewhat hyperactive life, I don't get much time to surf the net or watch TV but I do enjoy watching motor racing on the box, and I also get inspired by gardening programmes. Elaine and I love our garden and every time I see someone gardening on telly I can't wait to get out there and get my fingers in the soil.

Today, more than ever before, life offers so many exciting opportunities to keep both mind and body busy.

An old Maori lady once told me it was very good for the soul and she's right. There's something very therapeutic about getting out in the fresh air and creating your own personal Garden of Eden. It is good to slow down occasionally as well, although I must confess I've always had trouble sitting still for long.

I guess getting my pilot's licence wasn't what you'd call a goal until I became friendly with local flying instructor and former Air New Zealand pilot Phil Hooker, who now owns Bay Flight International Ltd at Mt Maunganui. Phil and I were both members of the model aircraft club and I taught him how to fly model aeroplanes. When he heard about disabled pilots in America using hand controls connected to the rudder pedal to fly proper planes he asked if I'd be interested in learning. Not being one to let a chance go by I naturally agreed and so he bought the gear and started giving me lessons. It took me 13 hours to fly solo and 50 to get my licence. Since then I've flown myself to a few speaking engagements and Phil's also transported me to one or two schools in his helicopter, which has been a thrill for both me and the kids I've gone to talk to. I hadn't ever really aspired to become a fixed-wing pilot but it was one of those occasions when opportunity knocked.

I've always believed in grasping any opportunity that comes my way with both hands. So many people are happy to just say, 'Oh well, maybe tomorrow', but, hey, tomorrow may never come and that's when you could end up regretting lost opportunities.

So, I believe we can inspire others and gain inspiration from many sources and a great range of people, from well-known public figures who have done great deeds or excelled in their career, to those that the world barely notices, but who face their difficulties with courage and dignity — people like Fay Goodall. By gaining a greater appreciation of who Fay was and what she was about and the challenges she went through in her life, I felt quite humbled and inspired. I also learnt not to judge people by their appearances. This world of ours has created a perception that if you're not perfect then you must be an idiot. People's perceptions or misconceptions are something I've had to contend with all my life as well and it is a subject I feel so strongly about that I'm devoting the next chapter to it.

Making a difference

~ You can do anything you want to. You just have to want to do it badly enough.

~ You don't have to succeed at everything, but at least have the courage to set yourself goals and then do your best to achieve them.

~ We can all inspire others and be inspired.

~ Your enthusiasm and passion can influence others. But so can just a look or a word.

~ Seek the inspiration of others. It only takes one person to make a difference in your life.

~ We all have stories ready to be passed on. Share your own story and try to hear others' stories.

~ Everyone should have dreams. If a goal is important to you, then go for it.

~ Life offers boundless opportunities. It is never too late to change your life, to have a good idea and run with it, to have a dream and turn it into reality.

3 perceptions and misconceptions

If losing my legs and my hair are the worst that ever happen in my life, then I feel truly blessed.

Legless — not hopeless

Despite having no legs I've never, ever thought of myself as disabled. In reality I consider myself more able-bodied than most people with legs because I've done more in my life than many will ever dream of doing, and I haven't finished yet. 'Disabled' is a label that has been stuck on me because we live in a world where we have to label things to make people feel more comfortable. I can understand that. I can understand the word 'disabled', so I can deal with that. But what I do have trouble with is the presumption that because I don't have legs I'm incapable of doing anything — of having dreams and goals and being successful at whatever it is I put my mind to.

For some strange reason there are even those who presume that because I have no legs I must surely be mentally retarded. It is true! I've been to restaurants where the waiter has completely ignored me and addressed all his comments to Elaine as if I didn't exist. Like: 'What would *he* like to drink?' Or else they presume for some strange reason

The only problem I have is with the presumption that because I don't have legs I'm incapable of having dreams and goals and being successful at whatever it is I put my mind to.

that because I have no legs I must therefore be deaf and so they feel the need to yell whenever they address me. Or else they touch me just in case I can't see. I sometimes get the feeling that people are too scared to shake my hand in case it drops off. Because I've lost both legs and most of my hair they're wondering what part of me is going to fall off next!

Earlier this year, after my trestles collapsed under me, I had to have a course of physiotherapy and, as often happens, the receptionist asked to see my Community Services card. She presumed that because I was in a wheelchair and had no legs I must therefore be a beneficiary. It never occurred to her that I might have a very successful business career. I'm also often asked to produce my ACC number because people see I have no legs and immediately jump to the conclusion that I am a recipient of Accident Compensation. So what do I say? I can't accuse such people of ignorance because that's just their perception; that's the world they live in. They think, 'Oh, he hasn't got legs. What can he do?' I could get indignant and abuse them but I just tell them, 'No, I don't have a community services card or an ACC number,' and leave it at that. I don't feel I should have to give detailed explanations, but hopefully just by saying no I will have changed their perception.

Many people find it hard to believe I'm married let alone a father and grandfather. Elaine likes to tell the story about the time she accompanied me to Vanuatu for a speaking engagement and everyone assumed that because we were together and had the same name we must be brother and sister. It just didn't occur to them that we might be husband and wife because over in Vanuatu people in wheelchairs are usually institutionalised. So people kept saying to Elaine, 'I feel really sorry for your brother,' and she kept telling them, 'He's not my brother, he's my husband.' They were quite shocked because they didn't think anyone with a perceived disability could have a wife. It was just unthinkable in their society.

One night after we'd been out for a meal there, Elaine went up to the counter to pay the bill and the receptionist said how sorry she felt for me. My wife retorted indignantly: 'Don't feel sorry for him. He's got a fabulous life. He's got a wonderful wife, a marvellous family, a beautiful home and a great career. He's one of the luckiest men in the world.' And she was right.

> *'Don't feel sorry for him ... He's one of the luckiest men in the world.'*

The fact remains, however, that when you're in a wheelchair there's always someone wanting to spoil your fun. Being a big kid at heart I love to ride on roller-coasters and all those fast, adrenalin-pumping rides whenever we visit fun parks such as Disneyland in the States, or Rainbow's End in Manukau City, here in New Zealand. But in many of those places they impose a minimum height restriction on many of the rides. It is aimed mainly at young children who are too skinny to fit safely into the frame. Now, because I have no legs I'm obviously not going to meet their height requirements but in every other respect there's not a problem. With my broad shoulders I'm definitely big and strong enough to sit in the seat and hold on tight, and once the safety bar is over me there is no way I'm ever going to fall out. Tough luck, Tony! They've made this blanket decision that if you're in a wheelchair or disabled or 'vertically challenged' like myself you can't go on and that's that. They reason that it is easier to make one rule for everybody rather than treat people in wheelchairs as individuals. It is so embarrassing and frustrating to queue for half an hour for a ride only to be told by some young attendant when you finally get to the front that you're not allowed on because you're too short or because you're 'disabled'.

> *Strangely, it is often left to those of us who are challenged in some way to be more tolerant of those who aren't.*

What do they know about my capabilities? Who are they to make such assumptions? Instead of doing everything they can to make life easier for people who are in some way physically challenged, all they do is make it harder. I think in the main they're motivated by fear. They don't know what it is like to be 'disabled' themselves and so they don't know how to handle such situations. They're afraid because they don't understand and it is left to those of us who are challenged in some way to become a little bit more tolerant of *them*. Having said that, I must confess I find it a virtue that's easier to preach than to practise! I don't like being told what I can or can't do. But I do understand people's fear, especially in this age where someone always has to be held accountable. We're always looking for someone to blame and that's especially so in the United States, where litigation is a way of life.

In the end, I got tired of having to argue it out at the head of the queue so now if I visit somewhere like Disneyland I go straight to the main office first and explain my circumstances and what rides I want to go on. They invariably give me the okay and ring through to the attendants to let them know that I'll be turning up.

A couple of years ago Elaine and I met the proprietor of Rainbow's End at a conference I addressed in Auckland. Not being one to let a chance go by, I told him how frustrated it made me to be told I couldn't do the fun things others took for granted when they entered his fun park. He sympathised but said it was not his fault. He told us he too couldn't believe how many restrictions the authorities imposed on disabled people going on his rides. Like preventing blind people from going on the roller coaster. Now why shouldn't a blind person go on a roller coaster? So what if they can't see? Most people prefer to keep their eyes tightly shut on rides like that anyway! The reasoning is that if anything goes wrong with a ride and it stops unexpectedly, if you're blind or disabled you won't be able to climb down. But as the proprietor pointed out, in the unlikely event of people being stranded on top of a ride like a roller coaster, everyone is taken down in a cherry picker anyway. As far as I'm concerned, if the thing was on fire I'd probably be the first down given my lifetime's experience of shinning up and down trestles.

It is the same when Elaine and I go to the local theatre. I can move around on my backside and am therefore not confined to a wheelchair, so we don't always choose to sit in the wheelchair section. But the minute staff see me arrive in a chair they start asserting their authority and telling us where we can and can't sit. If we try to sit downstairs near the front or away from an exit door they say: 'Oh, you can't sit there. What if there's a fire?' To which Elaine invariably replies: 'Watch him. Just watch him! If there's a fire he'll be out of here quicker than you and me!' And she's right. You'd be amazed how fast I can propel myself with my arms. I've had more than 30 years of practice so I should be good. In fact, my nickname at speedway used to be 'Cannonball' because of the speed with which I could roll away from a crashed car.

The saying 'Where there's a will there's a way' is true. You have to stick up for your rights and principles.

I have to admit there is one fun place where my lack of height has been an advantage, however. My son Lucas used to be very proud of the fact that I was the only dad who came within the maximum height restrictions in the McDonald's playground and now my grandsons are enjoying that fact as well. Only trouble is, being broad-shouldered I sometimes get stuck on the slides, which always causes lots of laughs among the kids, not to mention their parents and Elaine!

But joking aside, life isn't all beer and skittles when you're 'physically challenged' in some way.

When I was a signwriter I always used to say that whereas most people have 90 seconds to make an impression when applying for a job, I have only 30 seconds. The minute a prospective employer or client noticed I didn't have legs he or she immediately jumped to negative conclusions about my abilities and suitability. They had absolutely no idea what I was capable of; they just assumed that without legs I must be useless. So I had to get in there extra fast and show them how wrong their perceptions were, that just because I didn't meet their expectations in looks didn't mean I couldn't do the job, and do it well.

Don't let anything stand in your way

One of the reasons people assume my life must be extremely limited by not having legs is because of the perceptions they have of their own abilities. They come up to me and say, 'Oh, I could never do that' or 'Gosh, if that ever happened to me I'd just shrivel up and die.' Well, that's not how we do things in our family. Okay, so life's not fair, but it doesn't stop you achieving your goals. You've got to stop feeling sorry for yourself and get on with your life. You also have to learn to laugh at yourself. Spending a lot of time, as I do, on my backside I tend to see an awful lot of legs and I always joke that for the most part I'm glad I'm not wearing them. I've got some very good friends who fortunately take my warped sense of humour in the manner it is meant. At the beginning of summer when they put on shorts for the first time after a winter of wearing jeans I'll often look at their lily-white legs, sorrowfully shake my head and say: 'I had a pair like that once but I'm glad I got rid of them.' Actually one of my best mates is nicknamed 'Punga' because he's got really short legs with dark hair all over them, just like tree-fern stumps.

You've got to stop feeling sorry for yourself and get on with your life. And you've got to learn to laugh at yourself.

I don't believe life should be a fashion contest. Sure I could wear artificial legs if I wanted to. I'm sure the modern prostheses are a lot more comfortable and efficient than the ones I wore as a kid, and that I could look just the same as any other six-foot tall hunk! But I'm happy the way I am. People waste so much time worrying about such futile things. Who cares what they look like? So what if they're not wearing make-up or the latest designer clothes or Gucci shoes or their car's an old banger instead of a late-model Mercedes? The world isn't going to end because of it.

So you've got pimples or a pot belly or a protruding nose. That's your problem and no one else is going to care unless you make an issue of it.

People say to me: 'Gee, Tony, you're getting a bit thin on top,' and I say: 'Yeah, and I don't have any legs either, had you noticed?' What am I supposed to do? I'm losing my hair and I haven't got any legs — am I supposed to go and bury myself in a corner somewhere? Gosh, if those are the worst things that ever happen in my life then I feel truly blessed.

Life shouldn't be a fashion contest. Don't let how you look hold you back.

If you don't like who you are then fine, go ahead and make a change. If you're overweight, do some exercise. I carry a bit more weight than I should but I'm happy with the way I am. I don't know anyone who has said: 'I'm not going to have anything to with Tony because he doesn't have any hair and because he doesn't have any legs and because he's overweight.'

Honesty and humour

I can deal with the fact that I don't have any legs. Sure people stare at me but that's only natural. I'm different; that's fine. If I'm at a public swimming pool or somewhere like that people tend to look at me but that's due to their insecurity more than anything. They're scared because I don't have legs. Kids are so much more honest than adults. When they see me they just stare open-mouthed and their parents come up and grab them and push them away and say: 'Don't look at him, don't look at him,' and the kids yell, 'But look, look, he hasn't got any legs!' That's fine by me. Why stifle honesty? Having said that, I must confess I'm not always that honest when kids come up and ask me what happened to my legs. I was on the beach one day in Hawaii and a kid asked me and I told him a shark had got them. Another time we were sitting round the pool at our hotel and a youngster came up and asked me where my legs were. I looked down in surprise and said, 'Oh, I must have left them in the pool.' He spent the rest of the afternoon looking for my legs at the bottom of the pool!

When my kids were younger they used to bring their friends home from school and point to me and say, 'See, I told you he didn't have any legs!' I was a novelty to them but I think they were also proud of me and the fact that I didn't have legs. I'd like to think I was special to them rather than different. They've certainly got my sense of humour — they still insist on buying me socks for Christmas!

An honest, straightforward approach and a sense of humour go a long way in changing people's perceptions and coping with negative attitudes.

Once I helped rescue three teenagers from a dangerous rip in the surf at Papamoa when I was on lifeguard duty. There were two boys and a girl in trouble and being a normal red-blooded male I naturally chose to go out and bring the distressed damsel ashore in a rescue tube, leaving my mate, Warren Keenan, to save the two blokes. I managed to get the distraught girl safely into the shallows, but of course the water was still up to my neck and when she stood up and looked down at me and realised her heroic saviour didn't have any legs she promptly fainted! That caused many jokes among my mates, who reckoned I was responsible for almost as many accidents as I was rescues. This was a gross exaggeration I hasten to add, but it was all part of the camaraderie I enjoyed so much during my time with the Omanu Pacific Surf Club.

On another occasion, my friend Euan Cameron and I were taking part in an off-road truck race at Woodhill Forest, north of Auckland. Euan, who had an artificial leg, was driving while I was co-driver and navigator. We were speeding along Muriwai Beach at 120 miles an hour when we hit a rut and rolled end over end three times, finally coming to rest upside down. Although we weren't injured we had ruptured a tank and fuel was pouring everywhere so I yelled at Euan to get out quick. Unfortunately, his artificial leg was jammed between the accelerator and the brake pedal, so I had to quickly undo his prosthesis for him, whereupon he fell down and banged his head on the cab roof. I rolled out of the window and Euan followed me. He was hopping around on his one good leg, clutching his head and I was sitting in the sand beside the upturned truck wondering what to do next when another competitor went past and was completely shocked at the sight of us. He raced back to the pit area and told the officials to call for an ambulance urgently because there had been a horrific accident. He reported seeing one guy with his leg missing while another was buried up to his waist in sand! He couldn't understand why the officials didn't fly into a frenzied panic but, of course, they guessed immediately who he was talking about and therefore knew things were nowhere near as bad as they looked!

Elaine and I have to laugh sometimes at the way different people react to the fact that I have no legs. Some people stare, some look and then hurriedly turn away, while others go overboard fussing around me and wanting to push my wheelchair for me. In fact, my chair doesn't have handles so they would have a hard job but we realise they're only trying to help. We know it is done in good faith, but it always amazes Elaine because we've been together now for more than 25 years and she just never thinks of me as being disabled.

As Elaine says, showmanship does seem to come naturally to me:

'As far as Tony's current career is concerned I guess it helps that he's always liked being the centre of attention and entertaining people. He's always been a bit of a clown. I don't know why. Perhaps it has been a way of distracting attention away from the fact that he has no legs. Whenever we go out to dinner he is always the one who has everyone else in fits of laughter. He just loves to see people laughing and having fun and he especially enjoys being the one who makes them all laugh.'

Elaine and I share a positive attitude to how people react to me.

> 'Of course, because he doesn't have legs I've had to get used to people staring at us wherever we go but that's truly never bothered me and it doesn't bother Tony either. I must admit I've been shocked by the attitudes of some of the countries we've visited towards so-called disabled people. When we arrived at our hotel in Vanuatu and asked if they had a room with wheelchair access they assured us: "Oh yes, we've got a wheelchair room." But when I asked where it was they were quite perplexed by the question and replied: "At the hospital, of course." It obviously hadn't occurred to them in this supposedly enlightened age that hotels usually provide such a facility. Mind you, even when we've stayed at really flash hotels in some of the larger and so-called 'more civilised' cities in the world the wheelchair room inevitably looks out on the air-conditioning unit. There seems to be a mistaken belief that people with disabilities don't need a view. Or else they have twin beds because they assume people in wheelchairs can't possibly be married. Fortunately, we've both got a good sense of humour and we prefer to see the funny side of such ignorance rather than get bitter and twisted about it.
>
> 'Hopefully, Tony's able to change other people's misconceptions through his presentations and leave them a little wiser and more understanding.'

Pushing the limits with the Koreans

I always feel fortunate and blessed to be living in a place like New Zealand where I am able to pursue my dreams. In many Third World countries people who have accidents like mine or who have their legs blown off by landmines or whatever are more often than not just left to die, locked away in institutions, or given the most minimal assistance.

Korea is another country where the disabled have traditionally been locked away, out of sight and out of mind. Fortunately, there is a concerted effort currently being made to change that attitude and I'm grateful to have been able to assist in that process in some small way. I first featured in an hour-long documentary shown on Korean national television in 2000, and as I write this, my first book is about to go on sale there, having recently been translated into Korean.

Around the time I was writing *Race You to the Top*, a Korean television crew brought two disabled athletes to New Zealand to film them participating in a variety of outdoor pursuits and I was invited to join them. Through my business and sporting contacts I was able to help arrange some of the activities and I must say it proved to be a great experience. The Koreans were all fantastic people and we had a lot of laughs along the way.

Attitudes are improving. Even in countries like Korea where the disabled have traditionally been kept out of sight, some brave individuals are showing what is possible.

The athletes were a quadriplegic in his early twenties called Kim, who'd been involved in a car accident, and Yeung, 27 years old, a polio victim who had won a gold medal for swimming at the Paralympics. Little did these two guys realise what was in store for them when they arrived in New Zealand! Among other things, the producers had arranged for them to go white-water rafting, skydiving and sailing.

First, however, we all attended the Eve Rimmer Games in Whakatane, where Kim was told he was to compete in the ten-kilometre wheelchair race. Now the poor guy had never even been in a racing wheelchair before, let alone done a 10-kilometre race. He hadn't been a quadriplegic long so he didn't have a lot of strength in his arms and hands, but we soon learnt that once the producer had made up his mind nothing would deter him from achieving his goal. So off Kim went and he hadn't gone far when he hit the kerb and fell out of his chair, grazing himself quite badly, but the crew just picked him up and threw him back in, telling him to 'just keep racing'. It was really quite bizarre. They were running along filming him and he had blood pouring out of his arms and trickling down the side of his head! He ended up falling out three times and he was the last competitor to finish but at least he had the satisfaction of knowing he'd completed the race.

The Korean camera crew were really nice people but they were definitely demanding. By the end of the shoot Elaine and I were calling the producer 'One More Time' because that rapidly became his catch phrase. And if Kim had found the road race gruelling he was soon to find himself in a far more frightening situation. Skydiving! The idea was for Kim and me to be filmed tandem diving with a qualified parachutist. I'd actually done a tandem skydive once before so knew what to expect and was pretty excited about the whole thing but Kim was absolutely terrified.

At the Maramarua Skydiving Club the fun began. The Koreans' English was limited, but it soon became clear that the producer wanted to throw Kim out of the plane by himself. Because we thought he was joking we all roared with laughter, much to the producer's amazement. When we eventually realised he was serious, the instructor informed him he couldn't possibly allow Kim to do the jump alone, but the producer was equally emphatic and the ensuing exchange with an interpreter playing piggy in the middle was absolutely hilarious. In the end the instructor said it was a tandem dive or nothing and so the crew had to settle for that — much to the relief of poor terrified Kim, who didn't even have the strength to pull a rip cord! I'm afraid we didn't help matters by telling him we'd give him the nickname 'Splat', which was how he would have ended up if he had gone solo!

The next drama wasn't far away — it came when they were getting into the plane and tried to clip the cameraman in place. He argued vehemently that he didn't need clipping in, but because the plane for parachute jumps has no door it is an essential safety measure. Eventually he agreed to comply, after much discussion.

I waited on the ground while Kim did his jump and hurried over to meet him when he landed. The look of relief on his face said it all. He kissed me and hugged me and, in his broken English, said: 'Wery happy. Wery, wery happy to be back on the ground.' Fortunately for Kim, that was one occasion when the producer didn't insist he do it 'one more time'. He was saving that trick for the white-water rafting.

As with skydiving, I'd also been white-water rafting before. Through my signwriting business I'd become friends with Noel Rowson, who owns the Wet 'N' Wild Rafting Company in Rotorua, and I'd been down the Wairoa River in the Kaimai Ranges with him a few times. He arranged to meet us on the banks of the Rangitaiki River near Murupara early one morning. I took a couple of paraplegic mates along with me and the first thing the producer asked us to do was carry the raft down to the water ourselves. He was emphatic we had to do everything ourselves so there we were in our wheelchairs trying to hoist a huge rubber raft onto our heads and then wheel it down to the river. Yeung was walking along trying to steady it and after a bit of a struggle we finally made it.

They asked us to look scared but it was so hard not to whoop with excitement and cheer and laugh.

It was a spectacular day and after a bit of training on how to paddle we set off down the river with Noel and a cameraman in our boat and the producer and another cameraman in a boat behind us. Noel knew all the good places to film and sometimes we'd stop and let the other crew go past so they could then show us going over some particularly rough rapids. At one point they got out and filmed us from an overhead bridge. They asked us to look scared because they wanted the footage to show how challenging it was but that was really hard to do; we were having such a good time. These particular rapids were really fast-flowing and as we went down them there was water going everywhere, all over the boat, and it was so hard not to whoop with excitement and cheer and laugh. We had to try and sit there with a look of fear and trepidation on our faces but we just couldn't resist smiling a bit at the same time. When we got to the bottom of the rapids the producer was yelling: 'Go back. Go back. One more time!' Noel had lots of trouble trying to explain that we couldn't go back up the rapid because the water was flowing fast downstream.

Then he decided he wanted someone to fall in the water and I was probably the most, well, either gullible or stupid — I'm not sure which — so I said I'd go in. The water, just melted snow from the hills, was freezing, and I actually ended up falling out spontaneously the first time we hit a bump going down some rapids. I was floating down the river, bobbing up and down with rocks all around me. The water was rough and I was trying to hang onto my paddle but I had a life jacket on and being a good swimmer I was pretty confident. Nevertheless the unknown always worries you and it was extremely cold so I was quite relieved when the other guys finally managed to pull me back on board. The next minute, though, we heard from the bank those ominous words: 'One more time!' I ended up going in three times.

Next up on the filming schedule was sailing on Tauranga Harbour, on a boat called *Extreme*. The name says a lot about what the yacht was like: very light, fast and very, very frisky. So there we were out on the harbour in a strong breeze, with *Extreme* zooming along, up on her side, leaning way, way over, and poor old quadriplegic Kim, who'd never been on a yacht before, frantically trying to scramble across the deck!

The first time we went out was for a Wednesday night twilight race and we had a full crew on board, although we still had to do as much as we could ourselves. So we were pulling on the ropes and I was steering the thing and there was a helicopter up above with a cameraman filming us. It looked really impressive when the documentary went to air. We were getting the boat to lean right over and it was powering along and we finished either second or third,

I can't remember which. The next day the crew wanted to do some more filming so we took *Extreme* out again but this time with just a skeleton crew. Again they got us hauling sails up and down and steering the boat and I really enjoyed it — Kim and Yeung did too. Everybody had a great time and it was lots of fun — until the film crew wanted to get a bit more action into it and decided that someone should climb to the top of the mast. It still makes me hoot when I think of it! They had a bosun's chair, which is just a little sling that goes around your backside, and you get hauled up to the top of the mast on that. This time Yeung got the job because he still had the use of his legs, so two guys hoisted him aloft and I tell you what, he was the whitest Korean I've ever seen when he got back down.

I was floating around in the middle of the harbour as the yacht disappeared into the distance.

Next they decided someone should go overboard and you know who got the job — me! I waited until the boat was right up on its side and then I slid down to the lower side and went through the railing off the back of the boat. The idea was for Kim and Yeung to throw me a rope and pull me back on board as an act of friendship. So there I was getting towed behind the boat and they were pulling me in and I got about 2 metres from the stern when Yeung just looked at me with a funny smile on his face and let the rope go! The next minute I was floating around in the middle of Tauranga Harbour as the yacht disappeared into the distance. I can only presume the producer had pulled one of his usual tricks and told Yeung to drop the rope. It took about 10 minutes for them to stop the boat, turn it around and come back and get me.

My involvement with the Koreans was a tremendous experience and when the programme went to air it was one of the highest-rating documentaries they'd ever had on KBS Television. It was quite heart-rending because Kim was the main focus of the programme and they had his parents and a group of interviewers in the studio the night they showed the film, and everyone was crying as they watched the documentary, even the interviewers. Hopefully, it went a long way to dispelling some of the myths surrounding the 'disabled' in that country.

Since then the same crew returned to make another documentary about two blind people, one Korean and the other a Kiwi, climbing Mt Tarawera, which again rated extremely well. As I write this they're busy editing the footage of the Kilimanjaro climb, which is scheduled to screen in Korea some time in 2003.

Getting past the barriers

Although 99.9 per cent of my time is spent with able-bodied people — my family, my clients, my motor-racing friends — I must admit I do enjoy meeting other people in wheelchairs and particularly playing sport with them from time to time. It is really cool once in a while to be able to go into an environment where I'm the same as everybody else. I still like to play basketball whenever possible and it is a great feeling to be able to go out onto a basketball court with nine other people in wheelchairs and not be the odd one out. When I play wheelchair basketball the fact that I don't have any legs is not a disadvantage at all. I'm on a level playing field and that's a great feeling.

Sometimes when I'm playing basketball I'll fall out of my chair and Elaine and the kids will roar with laughter while onlookers around them will be shocked and horrified and gasp, 'Oh, is he alright?' But my family have grown up with their 'Daddy No-Legs' and they are used to my antics. So they laugh and think it is funny when something like that happens. This horrifies a lot of people because they think people like me should be wrapped in cotton wool! So many able-bodied people come up to me and say in sympathetic tones: 'I understand how you feel,' or 'I know just what you're going through.'

People are horrified when I tumble from my wheelchair. They think I should be wrapped in cotton wool.

In fact they've got absolutely no idea how I feel. How could they? Even those who've had similar things happen in their life have no idea what's going through my mind because we are all different and we all react differently to any given set of circumstances.

One of the most frustrating aspects of people's perceptions or misconceptions about 'disabled' people is the rules and regulations that are imposed on us by bureaucracy. In a world where litigation is becoming more prevalent and businesses are being made more accountable, this is in turn making life more difficult for the 'disabled'.

You have to find ways to overcome the difficulties that rules and regulations can impose.

Some airlines won't let disabled people fly because they need help going to the toilet. Is that right? They're still human beings, and paying passengers what's more, and as such they still have rights. I suppose I'm fortunate that I look able-bodied enough and I can head straight to the airline counter. The staff in airports I use regularly know that I take my wheelchair to the door of the plane and then jump out and go to my seat on my backside while the chair is stowed away in the hold. Some flight assistants are very good and pull my chair apart and store it at the front of the cabin. Sometimes someone will offer to bring me an aisle chair but I always decline. I don't want to use some horrible chair that's got a flag on top which says, 'Look at me, I'm disabled.'

One airline always wanted to stick me in a seat by the aisle the minute they saw 'wheelchair' on my ticket, but I prefer a window seat. Because I'm so broad-shouldered people tend to bump into me every time they go past if I'm sitting next to the aisle. And if I sit in the middle seat the people on either side of me are going to be squashed, but if I sit by the window I can turn around sideways and everyone's got enough room. One day this particular airline insisted I had to have an aisle seat and the woman at the counter wouldn't change it. I pointed out that I am usually seated by the window because in the event of an emergency the disabled are the last off the aircraft so they can be assisted by the crew. But it was all to no avail.

At the boarding gate, however, the attendant recognised me. I said: 'Look, they've put me in an aisle seat and you know an aisle seat's not going to be any good for me.' She just said, 'No problems, Tony,' and put me in a window seat and off I went. There's always a way! I try not to lose my cool but I do tend to stick to my guns and say, 'Hey, I'm the customer and this is what I want.' It is important that you make it clear what your requirements are, though, and then everybody understands and it makes life much easier. It certainly helps if you can retain your sense of humour throughout.

You can usually find a way around obstacles — if you assert yourself.

Much as I enjoy flying around the world it can nevertheless be fraught with frustrations for me in many ways quite apart from my seating arrangements. Like going through the metal detector at customs, for instance. Everyone has to go through and it beeps like mad and you see people hurriedly taking off their rings and brooches and belts and trying to hold their pants up with one hand while clutching their passports and airline tickets in the other. My wheelchair always gets the metal detector very excited; in fact I only have to go within 5 feet of the thing and it starts beeping loudly. Usually I go through anyway and stick my arms out and they wave a wand over me to make sure I'm not concealing anything metallic on my body. But occasionally, especially in the United States, they make me sit up straight and then feel all around me and stick their hands under my backside just to make sure I'm not concealing anything there. I tend to give them a sideways glance to warn them not to take too many liberties, but I tell you what, at end of the day I'm not going to get into an argument with big, tall, unfriendly, gun-toting American Customs and Immigration officers.

We once met a woman at the disabled games in Auckland who had no arms or legs. Despite her disability she was a very independent person who was doing the best she could to live as normally as possible without having to rely on others to do everything for her. But she found herself battling a lot of negativity and when we met her she was really upset because an airline had refused to allow her to fly to Auckland by herself because she couldn't get out of her chair unassisted. In the end she had to have someone with her who was dedicated to looking after her, not for her sake but to make the airline feel better.

I'm grateful I haven't had that thrown at me and I must admit that, on the whole, whenever I've come up against what I believe to be an injustice or an error of judgement I've found a way of fixing the problem.

If you don't ask, you don't get.

One day the firm of lawyers I deal with installed a new door that was too narrow for me to get my chair through. Someone always had to come and open up the second door for me and it was inconvenient, embarrassing and time-wasting. So one day I went along and got a new young lawyer and I told him I'd had enough. He suggested I write a letter of complaint, so Elaine and I wrote to one of the partners and for a while every time they knew we had an appointment they'd open both doors before we got there. Eventually they installed electric doors!

My determination to set and achieve goals is partly because people believe I can't do things. In my book 'can't' is not an option.

I suppose in some ways it is a reaction against other people's perceptions of what I can or can't do without legs that makes me even more determined to set and achieve my goals. Throughout my life I've had people tell me, 'You can't do that because you've got no legs.' I've always seen that word 'can't' as a challenge. People didn't believe me when I said I was learning tae kwon do. 'You can't do that,' they said. 'You've got no legs.' Well, not only did I prove I could do it but

I got a second-degree black belt in the martial art. So much for people's perceptions!

The world is full of opportunities, and we have endless choices — which is the topic of my next chapter.

Perceptions and misconceptions

~ We all have to battle others' perceptions and prejudices. People presume that because I don't have legs I'm incapable of having dreams and goals and being successful.

~ Don't let anything stand in your way. Remember that the saying 'Where there's a will there's a way' is true. Stand up for your rights and principles.

~ Don't let you own perceptions of yourself or people's views of you get in the way. Learn to laugh at yourself and get on with your life.

~ Life shouldn't be a fashion contest. Don't let how you look hold you back.

~ Honesty and humour really help in changing people's perceptions and coping with negative attitudes.

~ Attitudes are improving, and some brave individuals are showing the able-bodied world what is possible.

~ Assert yourself to get past the barriers, rules and regulations.

~ If you don't ask, you don't get.

~ Don't let other people decide what your limits are. Don't make 'can't' an option.

4 a wealth of choices

Success is a journey; the hard part is taking the first step — the rest is easy.

Seizing our opportunities

As a result of my accident I discovered very early on that we all have choices as to what we do with our life. We can either sit around feeling sorry for ourselves and waiting for the good times to come along, or we can actively go out there and make things happen. Many people think they don't have choices, that 'this is as good as it gets'. Nonsense. It gets far, far better, providing you believe in yourself and what you want to achieve. Look at me. I have no legs or feet and yet I consider myself one of the wealthiest people I know. And I'm not talking money here. I'm referring to the choices I have in my life because of my attitude and my self belief. I'm inspired by life and all that it has to offer and that in itself gives me choices.

We all have choices about what we do with our life. We can wait for the good times to come along, or we can get out and make things happen.

I think back 35 years to my first day home from hospital after my accident. I was a skinny little nine-year-old runt with no legs and for seven months I'd enjoyed round-the-clock care at Tauranga Hospital. I only had to click my fingers and I had nurses and doctors fussing round me. That first day home my dad put me on the floor in the lounge with some cushions to prop me up and then he went off to work. My brother and sister had gone to school and my mum was in the kitchen. All of a sudden I was all alone. Dead silence. After the hustle and bustle of hospital life it frightened me. I can clearly remember how upset and agitated I felt. I called out to my mother but there was no reply. I started to cry and then, like one of those roly-poly toys, I toppled over but, unlike them, I didn't bounce back. I was stuck and became even more agitated. So I started to roll, and I was rolling around the floor hitting my head and stumps on the door and the wall and the furniture and I thought, 'Hell, this isn't a very good idea,' so I began to drag myself along on my stomach, commando style. When I got to the kitchen, Mum was standing at the sink and I said, 'Mum, Mum.' She got a heck of a fright because she thought I was just lying back comfortably on my cushions. She was upset because she hadn't heard me calling out and I was obviously upset as well, but I realised there and then that just because my life had changed didn't mean the whole family routine had changed. Dad still had to go to work, my brother and sister still had to go to school, and Mum still had to do all the things mothers have to do.

> *Life wasn't always going to be fair to me, but it was how I dealt with it that was really going to make the difference, because I had choices.*

In those early days when I got home from the hospital my mother, who is only a little woman, would pick me up and carry me around the place but I soon got too heavy for that and so I learnt to do my own thing. I learnt to shuffle around on my backside and pretty soon I was propelling myself around with my hands faster than most people could walk. Then I was fitted with artificial legs, heavy steel things that were secured to my body with a metal band around my waist. I hated them. They really slowed me down and were always giving me trouble, as were my wooden crutches that had to support my weight plus the weight of the steel legs.

When I finally returned to school I got nicknamed Crippleson (a play on the word cripple and my surname, Christiansen). Kids can be very mean and horrible but I soon grew very hardened to all that sort of thing and, although it hurt to start with, I guess it was character building more than anything else. I had already discovered that life wasn't always going to be fair to me — in fact it had already been quite the opposite — but it was the way I dealt with it that was really going to make the difference because I had choices. I could have sat there and said: 'Why me? Why did it happen to me? Why couldn't it have been someone else?' But I suppose what it is really about is: 'Why *not* me?' I just had to find ways of coping with the down days and although they mightn't always have been the most admirable ways, at least I wasn't just sitting there passively taking all the insults kids threw at me.

From hobbling around on heavy metal legs with the help of crutches I started to get very big and strong, and if someone gave me a hard time it was nothing for me to pick up a crutch and give them a whack around the ears with it! Or else I'd swing one of my artificial legs around as the offender walked past and drop him like a brick. All of a sudden I became a person to be reckoned with rather than teased. That was me. Right or wrong, that was the way I dealt with it. These days you hear a lot about bullying in schools and how children who are a bit different in some way get picked on. Their parents often pop up on television shows like *Holmes* complaining about the injustice of it. My parents didn't have to worry about me, however, because I quickly learnt to fend for myself.

Other than using them as a defensive weapon (or offensive, depending whose side you were on) I never liked those artificial legs. I preferred to get around in a wheelchair or on my backside. When the time came for me to go to high school I was given three choices. I could go to Kaka Street School, which was really for the mentally challenged, which I was not; I could go to Tauranga Girls College, which was obviously supposed to be for girls (it had the advantage of being only a single-storeyed building); or I could go to the two-storeyed Tauranga Boys College, provided I wore my artificial legs. Being a born optimist and quick to grasp any opportunity that came my way I naturally voted in favour of the Girls College but alas, I somehow found myself at the Boys College instead! Ah well, I guess you can't have your own way all the time.

The principal of Tauranga Boys College, Norm Morris, said I was quite welcome to go there as long as I wore my artificial legs. He wanted me to look as 'normal' as possible; this was in the days before 'mainstreaming' became government policy in New Zealand. These days children with perceived 'disabilities' are encouraged to attend 'normal' schools and be integrated with 'normal' pupils. But back then they didn't have any other disabled or crippled students at the college.

Tauranga Boys College did make some concessions on my behalf, however. For instance it got the metalwork department to adapt a classroom chair so that I could be carried up the stairs to the second-storey classrooms when I was too tired to heave myself up there on my crutches and metal legs. A metal bracket was welded to either side of the chair so that a couple of my classmates could grab hold of them and carry me rather like an Indian rajah in a sedan chair. I quite enjoyed that and we used to have a lot of laughs. Most of the time, though, I got around on my artificial legs, which was very tiring and could also be quite hazardous, especially on wet days when the school's floors would become extremely slippery. Sometimes my legs would slip from underneath me and shoot out in different directions and I'd crash down on my backside. Not a pretty sight!

I realised that it doesn't matter what you look like — it's what you're like inside and what you do with your life that really count.

Although I was the only disabled pupil at Tauranga Boys College back then, it turned out that the school's rugby coach, Keith Empson, also had artificial legs. He'd lost both his legs after going through a hay baler as a youngster, and he taught me a lot about coping with a perceived disability. I'll never forget the day he was showing us how to kick the ball between the goal posts when the strap on his artificial limb broke and his leg instead of the ball went flying over the post. Obviously, we all thought it was hilarious to see his leg go flying through the air and then to watch Keith hopping frantically across the field to retrieve it. It made me realise that slipping over on wet floors wasn't so bad after all — and I came to the conclusion that it doesn't matter what you look like — it is what you're like inside and what you do with your life that really count.

The importance of self belief

One of the hardest things for most people is simply believing in themselves. I once read that the average 17-year-old in the Western world has been told 'No, you can't' 148,000 times. The challenge they face is that if they hear those negative words enough times they could start to believe them. Think about it. A kid comes home from school and goes to the fridge for a bottle of milk and ends up spilling it all over the floor. His mother says, 'Oh, you stupid little bugger! What did you do that for?' The next day he goes to school and does something wrong and his teacher tells him, 'Don't be so stupid!' Then he goes out onto the rugby field and misses a goal and his mates all yell, 'You stupid fool. What an idiot!' All of a sudden that kid starts to think he really must be stupid. Why? Because everyone keeps telling him he is. Well, we've got to start telling ourselves we aren't stupid, and that we are doing the best we can.

We need to remind ourselves that we aren't stupid, and that we are doing the best we can.

When our young grandsons come to see us they rush around touching everything the way kids do. Their mother says: 'Houston, don't touch that,' and Houston says, 'Why?' As happens so often with kids he gets told: 'Because.' And that's it. 'Because if you touch that lovely vase and it breaks then Nana will be really upset and we don't want to upset Nana, do we?' A child can understand that

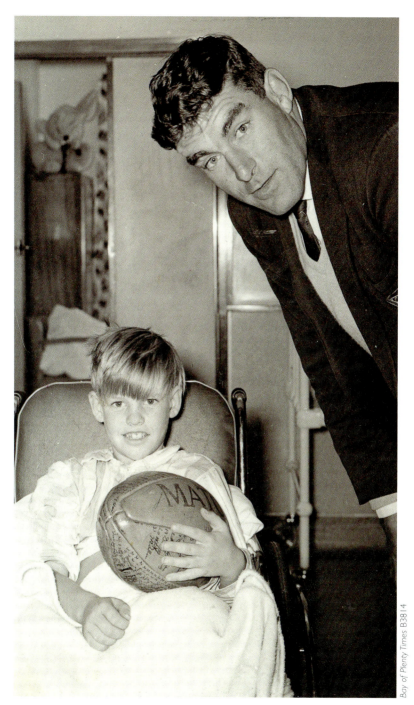

Colin Meads presenting me with the football
I still have today — a reminder in my office.

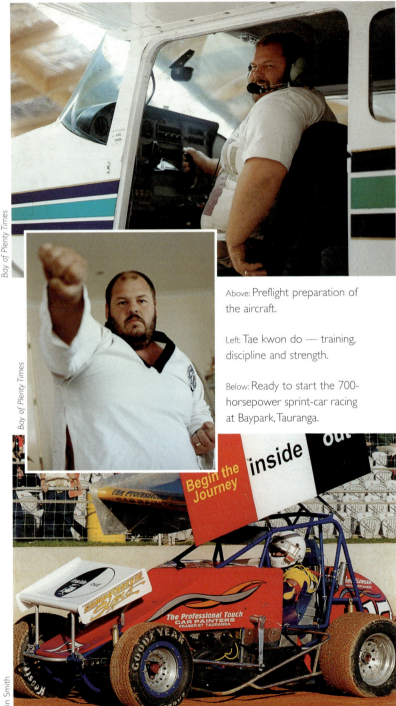

Above: Preflight preparation of the aircraft.

Left: Tae kwon do — training, discipline and strength.

Below: Ready to start the 700-horsepower sprint-car racing at Baypark, Tauranga.

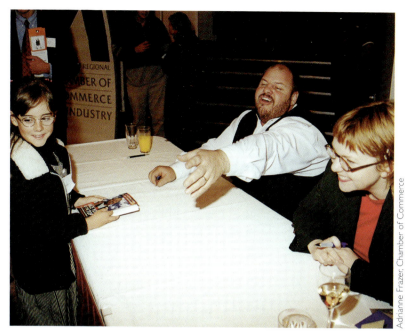

My niece Avalon at a book signing for *Race You to the Top*.

Speaking to 9500 people on the main platform at a Million Dollar Round Table conference in Toronto, Canada in 2001. An amazing experience.

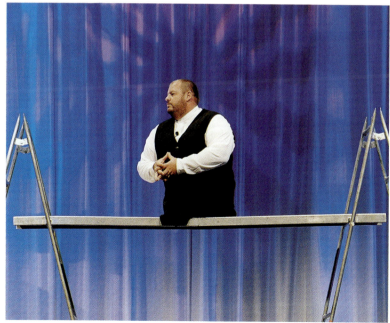

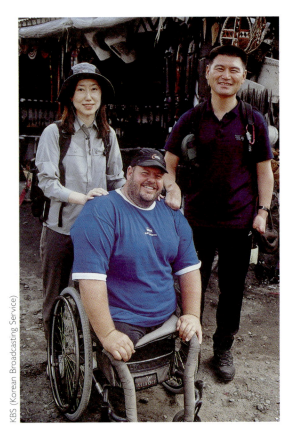

Soo Young, Hong Bin and I at the start of Mt Kilimanjaro.

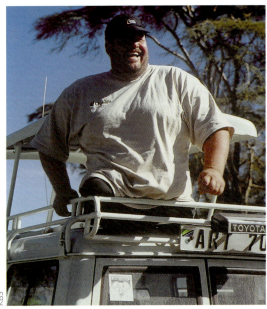

Atop the safari jeep in Ngorongorongo National Park, Tanzania.

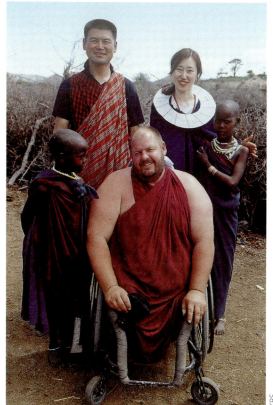

Right: Dressed in traditional Masai robes.

Below: The Korean Broadcasting Service documentary team with the Masai villagers, who taught us so much about the Masai way of life.

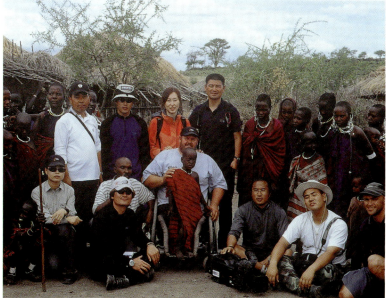

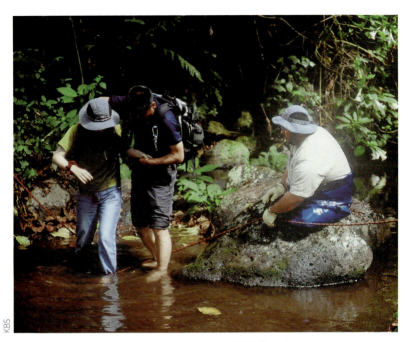

Soo Young and I crossing a stream at the base of Mt Kilimanjaro.

Crossing one of the many bridges on the lower trail with assistance from my porters, Godlisten and August.

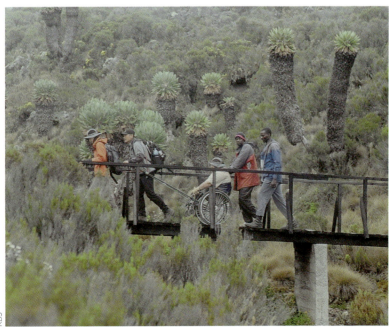

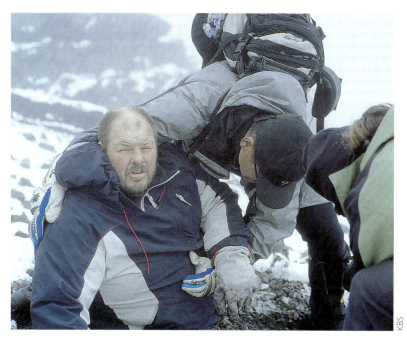

Above: We all need encouragement at some times in our lives. Here Hong Bin is helping me.

Right: On the way to the summit — it doesn't get much harder than this.

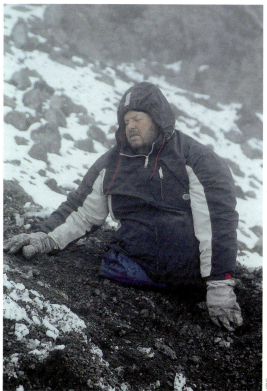

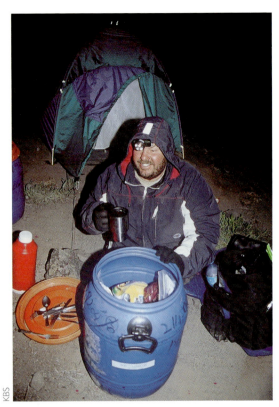

Left: Safely back at camp and thankful it's over.

Below: Ready to go home —going down is much faster than going up.

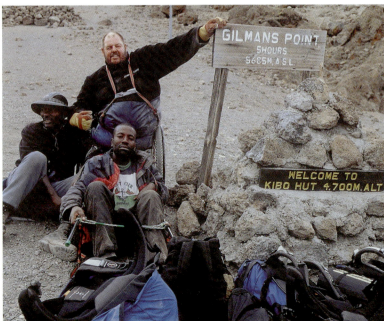

reasoning. But if it is not explained to them, you'll find a little bit down the track, when they're 10 or 12 years old, they'll do something wrong and when you ask them why they'll simply say, 'Because.' That's the only reason they've ever been given. They've been left to work things out for themselves and more often than not they've got hold of the wrong end of the stick in the process.

Having said that, I don't believe criminals should blame their parents for the way they behave. No matter what bad hand life has dealt them the choice is theirs whether they abide by the law or not.

I always say that success is a journey; the hard part is taking the first step — the rest is easy. You simply have to believe that success will come to you. Throughout my life I've got used to hearing such negative words and phrases as 'can't', 'shouldn't', 'couldn't', 'get real' and 'don't waste your time'. But such negativity makes me all the more determined to prove those people wrong. I firmly believe the maxims 'Success breeds success,' and 'If you hang around with losers that's all you'll ever be.' Despite what people think I have many choices as to what I can do with my life because of my attitude and my belief in myself.

Too many people today are lacking in self belief and if you don't like yourself you'll find that the life you'd really like to lead will pass you by because you haven't steered yourself in the right direction. In my opinion, as long as you seize every opportunity that comes your way and give it your best shot you're not a failure. You may not actually succeed at what you've set out to achieve the first time, but as long as you've at least tried then you're definitely not a loser. Instead, you've undoubtedly gained from the experience and will be so much wiser and more confident the next time you set yourself a goal. People tend to think that if they fail to

The hard part on the road to success is the first step. You simply have to believe that success will come to you and make the leap.

achieve their goal the first time round then they've got to start all over again from the beginning but that's not necessarily true. So often they've managed to reach the halfway mark to success and all they need to do is make a few minor adjustments to their strategy and then carry on from there. Anything positive you do in your life is not wasted. It all helps mould the person you are and the person you want to become.

If you grasp every opportunity that comes your way and give it your best shot you're not a failure. Anything positive you do in your life is not wasted.

Taking life seriously

Some people think success is all about money, while others say money doesn't bring you happiness. I have to say I know some very wealthy people who also happen to be very, very happy. I think what money does is allow you to have even more choices. I believe my wealth lies in the number of choices I have as to what I can do with my life. If money can help increase that number of choices then I'm all the richer for it. But, then again, I look at the Masai people in Africa who have very few choices and very little money and they seem pretty happy too. So it all boils down to your attitude and your self belief and how much you cherish life itself.

I believe one of the problems in this day and age is the fact that we're living in a throw-away society where everything and everyone is considered disposable. It is life in the fast lane, where people complain if they can't get you on the fax, Internet or cellphone 24 hours a day. If you don't get your meal at McDonald's in four minutes flat you get it free, and people go through life not knowing or caring a damn about the people they work alongside or the families who live next door. Fifty per cent, if not more, of all marriages fail, often because people give up far too easily rather than put in the effort needed to make a relationship work.

How often do you hear kids whining because they're bored? How can they be bored when they've got more opportunities and more playthings than ever before? They're subjected to so much advertising these days and they want everything they see. They have to have the latest high-tech skateboards and scooters worth hundreds of dollars whereas when I was a kid my proudest possession was a trolley my dad made me out of old lawn mower and wheelbarrow wheels along with some axles and bits of timber we got off my grandad. It would have cost $5 at the most to make and it gave me hours and hours of pleasure. It had ropes to steer with and it was a great thrill to go careering down hills in it. I remember taking the big wheels off it and replacing them with little steel wheels that made the trolley spin and slide all over the road because they didn't have traction. To me and my mates that was so much fun.

How wealthy you feel and what choices you think you have often depend on your attitude and self belief.

Then we'd go down to the creek at the back of my friend Paul Hodgson's place, where there were willow trees and a swamp and I learnt so much more there than if I'd just stayed home sitting on my bum watching television. We caught inanga and koura, tadpoles and frogs. We were out in the fresh air learning about nature and it didn't cost a cent. They were simple pleasures, but life was much simpler then. Those were the days (in this country at least) when sport was played for the glory of your country and personal pride rather than personal gain, before the word 'professional' entered the arena. Now our leading yachties are paid mega-bucks to sail for other countries. Then again, because we're living in a fast-paced, throw-away society sportspeople probably feel the need to make all the money they can while they're still able to. Look at the All Blacks. If one of them has a bad day he's thrown out and someone else takes his place. If they lose too many matches then everyone blames the coach and so he has to be replaced. It is not the sort of climate that encourages self-confidence.

There are knockers in all walks of life waiting to crush your dreams and crucify your self-confidence.

Self-doubt is more often than not a state of mind imposed on us by others who want us to fail because it makes them feel better about their own perceived inadequacies. In other words, we allow others to control the way we think about ourselves instead of having the courage of our own convictions. Can you imagine what people thought about the so-called 'insane ideas' the Wright brothers, Orville and Wilbur, nurtured when they were trying to make a machine that would fly? Small wonder they were labelled 'mad' and 'dreamers' but fortunately they were not deterred by other people's scepticism, but had the self belief and determination to pursue their dream and make it a world changing reality.

Don't give in to self-doubt. Ignore your critics and chase your dreams.

There are thousands of examples like those two brothers: Alexander Graham Bell, who invented the telephone; Karl Benz, who made the first petrol-driven car; Frenchman Joseph Niepce, who developed the first camera, which was later refined by American George Eastman; the list is a long one.

We all have a capacity for greatness within us; we just have to take all the opportunities — and sometimes the risks — to reach the next step of the journey towards being the very best we can be.

All the modern conveniences we take so much for granted today were once someone's dream or 'mad idea'. Then there are those who've inspired us in other ways, as we have seen in Chapter Two, in the fields of science, medicine, business and entertainment, as well as ordinary people who are not well known but whose examples are extraordinary. They are all people who've set themselves goals and worked hard to achieve them.

Remember, we can't get it right all the time. No one can. All the most successful people in the world have stories to tell of the failures and setbacks they suffered before they achieved their goals. The point is they didn't give up. They persevered and tried again, maybe in a different way or in a completely different direction, but they had enough self belief to know they would succeed in the end.

Since I became a professional speaker I've had the opportunity to meet many interesting people and some have even become good mates, such as well-known New Zealand comedian and television personality Mike King. I met Mike at a function I was addressing one night at which he was the MC. We had dinner together afterwards and having just listened to the story of my life he proceeded to tell me his — and it is a quite amazing tale, one that is typical of so many people who find fame and fortune. Mike is an example of the fact that success is rarely handed to you on a golden platter and it is definitely not something that can ever happen overnight. Most people struggle and work hard for years in an effort to turn their dreams into reality. More often than not they've put up with years of hard graft and financial deprivation to get there. Sometimes, as in Mike King's case, they've been hurtling along a downward path in life when something dramatic has happened to make them see the light and change course before it was too late.

Mike King is an example of someone who believed he had a choice and acted on it, something that changed his life.

Mike's defining moment came as a teenager after he'd got involved with a disreputable gang. He and his mate were the two youngest members and one night they were sent to a rival gang's headquarters with a couple of Molotov cocktails they'd been ordered to lob at the place. The leader of their gang drove them to the house involved and told them he'd be waiting at the corner of the street to whisk them away as soon as they'd done the dirty deed. So they threw the Molotov cocktails and their mate

69

promptly took off without them. Mike was convinced he was about to die and it was at that point that he asked himself: 'What the hell am I doing here? I'm going to die tonight and why? For whom? I'm risking my life doing something that is so ridiculous and lacking in meaning and on top of that my so-called mate has run off and left me.' Somehow he managed to escape before the rival gang could get their hands on him and he says that was his wake-up call in life. The choice was his whether he learnt from his mistakes or not. Fortunately for him and all his fans, he did.

Mike decided to do something more worthwhile and so joined the merchant navy as a chef. He became a good cook, which is something a lot of people don't know about Mike. One of the reasons he was invited to do TV commercials advertising pork was that he is well known as a funny man and the viewers were supposed to think, 'Well, if madcap Mike King can cook and cut pork like that, I should be able to do it too.' When he first started filming the ads it was his natural instinct as a former chef to make everything look professional, like on a cooking programme. The director kept having to stop him and ask him to try and act as if he didn't know one end of a carving knife from the other. Apparently it worked because Mike gets lots of feedback from people who've been inspired to try the recipes for themselves on the assumption that 'If he can do it so can I.'

Once in the navy and excelling as a chef, Mike's self-confidence grew, and so did his ambitions. He'd always liked making people laugh and he dreamt of one day becoming a full-time comedian. In fact the urge became so strong that about seven or eight years ago he reached another turning point in his life. He had to decide whether to stay with the security of a job he was good at and that paid well, even though it didn't really satisfy him, or take a punt and try something less secure but dearer to his heart. He chose the latter and despite having a wife and young family to support he decided to try forging a new career for himself on land as a comedian. Mike's passion was so strong that he was prepared to take risks to achieve his goal. He began entertaining on a part-time basis and now is one of New Zealand's best-known comedians, having hosted numerous comedy series, starred in commercials, and appeared at comedy festivals all over the world. As if all that's not enough, he now also runs his own celebrity speaker's agency and a travel agency as well! He's a great example of someone who overcame the odds and worked hard to achieve success.

Use it or lose it

Unlike Mike, I don't really know when my defining moment was. Perhaps it was coming out of the intensive care unit at Tauranga Hospital as a nine-year-old with no legs and thinking, 'Well, this isn't very good, but I shouldn't just feel sorry for myself.' Or it could have been when I was finally allowed home seven months later and I realised the world wasn't going to revolve around me any more and I had to fit back into family life and learn to do my own thing again.

I believe that the day I had my accident I could quite easily have died but it wasn't my time. No one ever knows when their time might be up, which is why we owe it to ourselves to grasp every opportunity that comes our way. So many people have the opportunity to pursue their dreams or achieve their goals but for one reason or another they choose not to take it, which is sad because one day that opportunity will be lost. One day it'll be taken away, so use it or lose it.

The world won't wait for you. Grab every opportunity that comes your way.

Don't settle for mediocrity either. Think about it. What makes people successful? What makes New Zealand's gold medal winning shot putter Beatrice Faumauina successful, for instance? The fact that she's not going to accept a lesser level for herself. For some reason, she didn't even make the top six at the Sydney Olympics but she didn't just throw in the towel and give up competitive sport. She had let herself down and she was determined to prove to both herself and her country that she could do better. And she did. Two years later she won gold at the Commonwealth Games in Manchester and people loved her all the more for her courage and perseverance. Likewise, everyone thought Kiwi swimmer Toni Jeffs was over the hill at thirty. Not so! She was completely focused on her goal, putting in all the hours of hard training that makes a champion swimmer and she was rewarded with a bronze medal at Manchester, her second bronze at a Commonwealth Games. She'd also won one four years before at Kuala Lumpur. Fortunately, she hadn't taken heed of the knockers and sceptics, who believed she should have retired from competitive swimming, and by achieving her goal she had the added satisfaction of proving them all wrong. What do other people know about our abilities and our determination to succeed? Many of us don't even know our own limits and limitations ourselves. But at the end of the day we are the ones who decide what we will or won't do — not somebody else.

Sportspeople like Beatrice Faumauina and Toni Jeffs showed what can be achieved with courage and perseverance.

My ability to learn tae kwon do and progress enough to teach the martial art, despite obvious impediments, has always been a good lesson for my young pupils. They can see that they shouldn't listen to people who try to tell them they haven't got what it takes to achieve their goals, whatever they may be. I must confess they learn one or two other slightly more painful lessons as well. I used to really enjoy training the 12–14-year-olds and we'd often do free sparring, where they'd come up to me and do no-contact kicking and things like that. I'd block their shins with my forearm and because my arms are so strong they'd invariably come off second best. I used to always make them wear two shin pads and initially they'd laugh at me, as they thought I'd be an easy target, but after a while they nicknamed me 'No Control' because they'd end up limping away in pain. It became a running joke — when any kid was seen limping out of the hall people would say: 'Oh, free sparring with Tony tonight, were you?'

A couple of years ago I was invited to give a Saturday lunchtime presentation at the New Zealand Independent Timber Merchants' (ITM) conference, which was being held in Brisbane. Elaine and I were invited to spend the whole weekend there and on the Friday afternoon we went on a cruise with some of the delegates for a barbecue on Stradbroke Island. We got to meet a lot of different people on the boat and most of them didn't know I was to be a guest speaker. I didn't enlighten them because I didn't want to spoil my surprise entrance at the start of my presentation. Anyway, heading back to Brisbane after the barbecue I starting talking to a guy at the back of the boat and he told me a fascinating story about how he and four team-mates had represented New Zealand in speed ice-skating at the Winter Olympics nearly 10 years ago. Now, how many people knew we'd ever sent a team of ice-skaters over to the Winter Olympics? I certainly didn't. As far as I know there are no longer any speed skating rinks left in New Zealand, but 12 years ago a team of Christchurch guys skated for hundreds of thousands of hours just going round and round a rink in a bid to be the fastest in the world. And they made it.

> *The story of the New Zealand ice-skating team is an incredible one of setting goals and achieving them through sheer determination, hard slog and self-motivation.*

If you've ever seen that neat movie *Cool Runnings* about the Jamaican bobsled team then you're going to enjoy this story as told to me by Tony Smith of Wellington:

> *'As a kid growing up in Christchurch I used to go to the public sessions at the ice-skating rink and one night I saw a visiting Australian team racing against a New Zealand team. The idea of*

speed skating appealed to me so I saved up to buy a pair of speed skates and it wasn't long before I was hooked on the sport. There weren't many ice rinks in the country in those days but in winter we could often skate outdoors at a place called Lake Ida.

'Anyway, back in the mid to late 1980s I competed in the national skating championships and also competed in Australia as well. In 1987 it was announced that short-track speed skating was to be included as an official demonstration sport at the Winter Olympics in Calgary, Canada, the following year with the understanding that if it was a success it would get full medal status at the 1992 winter games. A couple of New Zealand guys decided to go over to Canada to try and qualify. From memory I think the top 32 would get to compete and they finished thirty-third and thirty-fourth. But despite just missing out they came back to New Zealand full of enthusiasm and the following year the speed skating event was a great success at Calgary. We knew there could be a chance of competing in the Olympics but round about this time I decided it would be best if I retired from the sport. Not only was I starting a new job, I was also getting married and building our first house, all in the space of a few months. I still kept in contact with my skating friends but at that time the Olympics were the last thing on my mind.

'My interest was rekindled a couple of years later, however, when I learnt that the world skating championships were to be held for the first and only time in the Southern Hemisphere — in Sydney. In order to qualify for the 1992 Winter Olympics, competitors would have to be placed high at the world champs. It was a challenge I couldn't resist! Although we had some very talented individual skaters in New Zealand at the time we decided to target the relay event, a 5000-metre race involving teams of four skaters. We'd raced the event at our own nationals and it was always a very competitive race between the local clubs — there was a prized trophy to win.

'After the decision was made to go for it we approached the head of the University of Canterbury's sports science department, Paul Carpinter, and told him of our plan. He did some research based on where we were at compared to the rest of the world and what we would have to do to get to the top. Interestingly, at our second meeting he advised us that he didn't think we had enough time to prepare but in hindsight I'm sure this was a bit of a scare tactic to motivate us. And it worked! Training wasn't just on ice. There was cycling (for endurance), weight training (for strength) and sprint training (for speed). We did it all. Whatever it was going to take. Our performance and improvements were monitored to make sure we were making the required gains.

'The world champs in Sydney arrived and we were looking for a top eight place to get one of the spots at the winter games. We didn't have a big budget and we stayed at a camping ground till the day before the competition started, which was when the organisers started paying for the competitors to stay in a hotel. From memory there were 16 teams entered for the relay, including all the big countries, USA, China, Canada, Holland, Great Britain, Italy and France. It was very daunting. It meant there would be four heats of four teams, and first and second from each heat would move to the semi-finals, which of course meant the top eight.

'We drew Italy, China and USA. We had never even raced these guys before, let alone in a world championship event, but we did have a few things in our favour: we were the underdogs and we had done the work. We finished second in the heats, second in the semis, and second in the final. We were on our way!

'The Olympics in Albertville, France, in 1992 were amazing. Here I was at an Olympic Games after all but giving up the sport, *and short-track speed skating no less. The sport was so small in New Zealand that nobody even knew we were there apart from friends and family. I think at that stage there were only two rinks in New Zealand where we could train. Competitors from other countries would jokingly ask if we'd remembered to turn out the lights when we left New Zealand but we took it all in good part. We were making a difference and we had the sport talking. All the other teams' coaches would come down to the training sessions to watch us train.*

'At this time the world record for the 5000-metre relay was 7.22 minutes held by the Dutch. We won our heat in 7.21 and were placed second in the semi-final, beating Australia and France in 7.20. If somebody had asked me a month earlier where we'd come if we could do it in 7.20 I'd have said first. As it was we skated 7.18.91 in the final and finished fourth! We missed getting a bronze medal by a mere 0.7 of a second!

'I can remember gliding around the ice watching the three other teams celebrating and waving their flags and thinking, "Rewind the tape; this isn't how it was meant to happen; what went wrong?" At this stage I was meant to be climbing over the barriers and up into the stands to hug my wife, Joanne. I looked over and saw her standing right at the front holding a rose she had planned to give me as I triumphantly skated past her to go to the changing rooms. I sat down at the side of the rink gazing out onto the ice wondering how I could possibly walk past her now. I felt I'd let her down so badly. I sat there putting on my tracksuit and contemplating my next move and, to make matters worse, when I looked up the officials were rolling out the red carpet and setting up the medal dais for the presentation ceremony. I just wanted a hole to open up and swallow me. I had to get out of there so I got up and started walking towards the exit. I could hardly look in Jo's direction. As I went past her she

reached out with the rose and all I could say in a quivering voice was, "Sorry, honey." Definitely not the best day of my life!

'So where did we go wrong? I'll tell you. After the semi-final we had one hour until the final. We were in the changing room sharpening our skates and doing all the usual pre-race stuff and then we started talking about what medal we would get. I can even remember how we narrowed down the result. Korea: too strong, too fast. They'll win it. Canada: last three times we raced them we won twice. Japan: we beat them in the heats, we'll beat them here. We gave ourselves the bronze medal, or maybe even the silver, before we had skated a lap. We were up there on the dais even before the gun went off and as it turned out we weren't even in the placings. Korea did indeed win, Canada came second and Japan third. We'd been good enough to win a medal that night but we'd focused on the end result rather than how we were going to get there. We'd talked ourselves out of it. It was a hard lesson to learn but as a result one of the team sayings became: "The pain of discipline is far better than the pain of regret."

'Our first trip to Albertville confirmed we lacked experience and cohesion as a team. We were five individuals with different ideas on how much and what type of training we should be doing and we lacked the discipline to listen to our coach and work as a team. Over the next few months with the aid of hindsight and help from a great team of support people we learnt to think differently. No longer was there such a thing as doing a time trial and then coming off the ice saying: "Not bad but I could have gone faster if..." Basically we learnt to "pay the price".

'Twelve months later at the world championships in China we won the relay in the world record time of 7.10.95. This meant we would travel to the 1994 Winter Olympics in Lillehammer, Norway, as one of the favourites. As it turned out, everything that

could go wrong did go wrong and we finished up being disqualified in the B final after some terrible crashes, but this time I had no regrets because, unlike Albertville, I wouldn't have changed anything I did. As a team we all gave the best we could but it just wasn't good enough on the night. That defeat was a lot easier to accept than the one in 1992.

'We actually saw the movie Cool Runnings while we were in Lillehammer and we were amazed at how similar it was to our own story. Just like the Jamaicans we had little funding. We wore home-made uniforms and paid for our own airfares and accommodation to get to qualifying competitions. We had only one pair of skates each, which meant no back-up if they were stolen or damaged in training. I was the only one holding down a full-time job. The rest of the team worked part time in between training. Money was sparse and so was sponsorship but we were all passionate about our goal of wanting to win an Olympic medal. Even the ending in Cool Runnings was similar to our experience at the Lillehammer Olympics except that in our case we had proved ourselves in China the year before and were world champions and world record holders and therefore the favourites going into the Olympics. In the build-up to Lillehammer our team psychologist had taught us to focus on what we could control: our performance and attitude and visualising a positive outcome. "Control the controllables," we were told. Unfortunately, everything that went wrong on that day was influenced by someone else and out of our control.

'But despite the hard work and heartaches they were good times and we had a lot of fun. We were amazed at the support we received from New Zealand once we were competing at the Olympics. One of the most valuable parts of our build-up to Lillehammer was having funding for a team masseuse, dietitian and psychologist. The fact that they were outsiders from our close-knit *skating contacts, not to mention experienced people who had trained and worked with other successful teams, forced us to stand back and take more notice of their advice.*

'For me, one of the important lessons I learnt before it was too late was that at our level you still needed to try and maintain some level of balance in your life. We were completely focused on our dreams and training twice a day, six days a week. I had a very supportive employer but was still working full time between competitions, and my wife and I became like ships in the night. Our team psychologist suggested we devote one night a week to spending some quality time with our partners, otherwise they wouldn't be there for us when the Olympics were all over. We were all in relationships at the time and it was a timely wake up call. My wife will confirm that it is no fun being a "sports widow" as she termed it. As much as your partner wants you to be successful and believes in your dreams and abilities, it is no fun being the one left behind when you travel overseas and it can be a very lonely existence for partners.

'Our team broke up in 1994. Since then there have been two more Winter Olympic Games, one in Japan and the other in the United States. In both those games we only had one competitor in individual events. Unfortunately, the sport has not been able to go on from where we left off and we have not sent a relay team to any overseas competitions.

The New Zealand ice-skaters' success had a lot to do with attitude: believing they could be as good as teams from the great skating nations. It is this sort of positive thinking that I will discuss in the next chapter.

A wealth of choices

- Life isn't a dress rehearsal. We only get one crack at it so we owe it to ourselves to make the most of every opportunity that comes our way.

- We all have choices about what we do with our lives. We can wait for the good times to come along, or we can get out and make things happen.

- The hard part on the road to success is the first step. You simply have to believe that success will come to you and make the leap.

- The most successful people in the world have stories to tell of the failures and setbacks they suffered before they achieved their goals. They didn't give up.

- If you give everything your best shot but don't succeed, you're not a failure. Anything positive you do in your life is not wasted.

- The choices you think you have depend on your attitude and self belief.

- We all have a capacity for greatness; we just have to take all the opportunities — and sometimes the risks — to reach the next step of the journey towards being the best we can be.

the power of positive thinking | 5

If you don't enjoy it,
don't do it.

Getting the most out of life

People often ask me what I think I would have done with my life had I not lost my legs as a child. Who knows? One thing's for certain, though. I wouldn't have been tied to a job I didn't enjoy and I would still have had the same energy and determination to succeed, because that's the way I am. The train accident may have taken away my legs but it didn't take away my heart and my passion for life. I've always had an inquisitive and adventurous nature. Even before my accident, as a very young toddler, Mum says I was forever climbing over the fence into the neighbour's property. I was always pushing the boundaries and I'm still doing it today. It is all about attitude and the power of positive thinking.

In my presentations I always stress the importance of having a positive attitude to life. Some people will try to tell you that hard work is the key to success and others maintain the most important ingredient is knowledge. I was helping my grandson, Houston, with his homework one day and for some reason he had to number all the letters of the alphabet from one to twenty-six. I decided to do a little experiment. I added up the values of the letters

We only have one thought at a time and the choice is ours whether it's a positive thought or a negative one.

that spell HARD WORK and found they came to 98 per cent. Then I did the same with the word KNOWLEDGE and that came to 96 per cent. I then added up the corresponding values in the letters ATTITUDE and, what do you know — they totalled 100 per cent! Then I thought about how people often tell you to aim for more than 100 per cent if you want to succeed, so I did a quick count on the word BULLSHIT and that equalled 103 per cent! So don't waste your time striving for things you can't possibly achieve. There's no such thing as 110 per cent — 100 is all you need. You either give something your best effort or you don't, and if you do then it is always going to be 100 per cent. And that means having a positive attitude in everything you do.

A lot of people don't appreciate what a wonderful gift life itself is. It affords so many exciting opportunities and choices and we never know what is going to be on the next terrific page in our book of life. We're here on Earth for such a short time and it seems a crime to waste that gift and all those opportunities, but so many people do. How many people do you know who are doing the same thing today that they were doing ten years ago? They're stuck in limbo. I know people who've been dead for ten years — they just don't know it yet! Because they've been doing the same things year after year. But life changes every day and we owe it to ourselves to keep up with those changes. I'm not suggesting you change job or move house every year, but you should be availing yourself of every opportunity that comes your way. In other words, you should be getting the most out of this precious commodity called life. Let's face it, we never know what's going to happen tomorrow. We don't have a crystal ball and we don't know what's around the corner. It is all very well to keep putting things off till another day, but none of us knows for sure that there'll be another day.

Look at the people in New York. Never in their wildest imaginings would they have envisaged the horrible events of 11 September 2001 when terrorists flew two planes into the Twin Towers, killing thousands of people. That one act changed the world in so many ways. It made us more aware of man's inhumanity to man and it made us realise how temporary everything is on Earth. It made a lot of people appreciate their families more, and here in New Zealand we were all grateful that we lived in a little country far away from such horrific acts of violence. Except that for Elaine and I, we weren't that far removed from it because our daughter Danie happened to be living in New York at the time. We were awoken at four o'clock that morning by her phone call and she was screaming down the phone: 'Dad, Dad, they've flown a plane into the Twin Towers.'

She was working as a nanny on Rhode Island, two and a half hours' drive from the centre of New York, but she could see the smoke from there. So one minute she was having a wonderful working holiday and the next minute she was witnessing a tragedy that shocked the world. She was lucky and so were we. So many other tourists chose that morning to visit the Twin Towers and their families never saw them again. It was still very traumatic, though, and Danie, who'd originally planned to stay there a year, changed her mind and came home four months early. Now she's a nanny here in Tauranga.

You can't let sad events stop you, however. Life must go on and, sure, it isn't always smooth sailing. I learnt that lesson very early in life. But with the right attitude you can overcome the bad times and the sad times and all the negative things that happen along the way. The important thing is not to harbour negative emotions, such as bitterness, hatred, jealousy or envy. Don't bear grudges. Life is too short.

I read that a man had lost his teenage daughter in a terrible accident involving a lot of other teenagers at a party. A car had ploughed into a group of kids injuring many of them, and this man's daughter had died as a result. But the grief-stricken father said he didn't hate the young woman who'd been driving the car because, as he put it, 'Life is too short to go around disliking people.' What a wise man. What a pity more people don't share that attitude. It is not easy to forgive those who've wronged us, but if you go through life bearing grudges and feeling angry and bitter about something you're only prolonging your own suffering. You have to learn to put the bad times behind you and move on.

Sorting out your attitude

I strongly believe that to be successful in your business life you must first be successful in your personal life. So many people go through life carrying 'baggage' around with them, doing things they don't want to do, being in relationships they don't want to be in and working at jobs they don't enjoy. My motto is: "If you don't enjoy it, don't do it," because you're not going to give it your best shot and therefore it is a pointless exercise. Employers want successful people working for them and, as I see it, if employees aren't successful in their personal lives then they're not going to be much use career-wise either. If people bring all kinds of personal baggage to work with them each day it is probably going to take them four or five hours just trying to clear their heads before they can even start to do the job they're being paid to do.

Bad, sad and negative things can be overcome. Don't harbour negative emotions, such as bitterness, hatred, jealousy or envy. You've got to move on.

You know what it is like if you've had a row with your partner and the atmosphere at breakfast is icy or volatile. Or the kids have hogged the bathroom and you're running late or the paper boy or girl has forgotten to deliver your morning paper. Or perhaps you blew all your money at the casino at the weekend and now you can't afford to put food on the table let alone pay your bills. Or you went on another drinking binge last night and you're nursing a giant hangover and, what's worse, you can't remember what you did and whom you did it with. Whatever the problem, the chances are you're going to spend a large part of your day preoccupied with feeling angry or hurt or just downright sorry for yourself instead of concentrating on your work.

In other words, you're short-changing your employer and short-changing yourself as well.

You need to sort out your own backyard before you go to work. Don't take whatever challenges you have in your personal life through into your workplace because that's going to affect your productivity and therefore your usefulness to your employer. 'Easier said than done,' I hear you cry. Okay, so no one said life was easy. You've got to work at it. People have to learn to deal with their problems and move on. Life is too short to go around with a chip on your shoulder. Everybody has baggage, but it is how you deal with it that counts.

> *Everyone has negative baggage, but it is dealing with it positively that counts.*

If you're going through a bad patch and feeling sorry for yourself you'll find the more you dwell on the negative aspects of your life the deeper you'll sink into the mire of depression and self-pity. Your doctor may prescribe antidepressants but what's really called for is a change of attitude. It is all to do with the way you think about things: positively or negatively. For instance, you can get up in the morning and feel really crappy and think life sucks. It is a terrible day, pouring with rain, and you don't want to go to work. How many people get up feeling like that every morning? Heaps. How much better to get up, throw back the curtains and go 'Ooowhee, what a great day! I've got so much to look forward to. Sure I've got to go to work but, hey, it is only for eight hours. And okay, so it is wet, but that doesn't matter because it is not going to stop me doing the things I want to do.' Think about it. When it rains most people get out of their car and get their feet wet. When I go out in the rain I get a wet bum! But does it matter? Not to me it doesn't. It is all about acceptance of who you are and what you are and then moving on from that. I really think most people don't accept themselves. As I said at the beginning of this book, I guess if I wanted to I could just sit around in my wheelchair all day, every day, feeling sorry for myself and asking why was it me who got run over by a train? But I don't because that's not my style.

The former president of the National Speakers Association in Australia, Doctor Terry Paulson, provided me with a testimonial once that I think says a lot about the power of positive thinking. He wrote:

Tony Christiansen is enthusiasm, drive and joy bundled together in one unusual but inspiring package no audience will be able to forget. Optimism is not Polyanna thinking; each person must earn it by building a track record of overcoming obstacles on the way to excellence. When you hear Tony's story and see him soar on stage without legs or wings, you leave realising no excuse should ever stop you from doing anything less.

Direct your energy into positive thoughts

Like so many people who've had a brush with death I learnt at a very tender age what a fragile hold we have on life. How many times have you heard people recovering from cancer say: 'Having such a close call taught me to appreciate life so much more and to cherish my family and friends and all that I've got'? Life is too short to waste precious moments worrying about what might have been. I might not have legs but I absolutely love life and enjoy every minute of it.

People often ask me why I don't wear artificial legs. I suppose that if I did I'd look more 'normal' and wouldn't attract so many stares. But what's normal? I tried wearing prosthetics in my younger days and I found them cumbersome and uncomfortable. My stumps tend to tingle all the time because of the nerve endings being cut and I found that artificial legs merely exacerbated the sensation. I feel much more comfortable without them. Sometimes if I get too hot or maybe a bit agitated then my stumps pulsate and I'm really conscious of them. I don't know why they do that and I don't particularly want to know. It is just something that happens occasionally and it is usually short-lived.

I get on with what I'm doing or else I think about something else and the sensation goes away. It is a bit uncomfortable but it doesn't cause me any great distress.

In fact, I'm very fortunate to be able to say I've never had any real pain in my stumps at all. Once when I was a kid I had what's called a 'phantom limb'. I felt like I had an itch in my foot that I wanted to scratch. That was when I regained consciousness six days after having both legs amputated and it was when I went to scratch my foot that my mother broke the news to me about my legs. The last time I wore my artificial legs was about three months after I'd started going out with Elaine, 25 years ago. She'd never seen me with them so one day I thought I'd impress her. She was waiting for me in the lounge as I struggled to get them on in my bedroom. I finally managed to stand up on the ungainly contraptions and clumped my way unsteadily down the hall. I was trying desperately not to lose my balance and fall flat on my face as I flung open the lounge door and leant, in what I hoped was a nonchalant fashion, against the wall. You know, the sort of pose John Wayne or Clint Eastwood would adopt in the movies when trying to impress a girl: 'A man's got to do what a man's got to do.' It always worked for them. But instead of being impressed my future wife merely roared with laughter and said, 'Take them off, you look so stupid!' So much for the movies. It was probably around that time that I learnt it was much better to just be yourself and that looks weren't really that important. Anyway, after that I threw the legs in a cupboard and never wore them again. I'll let Elaine tell the story of what happened to them after that:

> *'I think Tony was secretly relieved that I preferred him without artificial legs because they were far from comfortable to wear and he's always been much happier getting around on his hands and backside — and quicker too. Anyway, the legs cluttered up the place for years until we were moving house one time and decided*

to have a big clean-out. We were piling junk onto a trailer and the artificial legs got thrown on as well and taken to the dump. They were metal legs that stood up by themselves, rather like a suit of armour. In those days an old Maori lady lived in a little house alongside the dump and you had to pay her something like 50 cents to tip your rubbish there. Well, they say one man's trash is another man's treasure and that was obviously the case with Tony's legs because the next time we went to the dump there they were standing proudly on the woman's porch with beautiful flowering shrubs growing out of them. She was using them as plant pots! We thought that was rather a nice ending for them and they were certainly a lot more use to her than they'd ever been to Tony.'

I've never worried too much about what I look like. Worry is a terrible emotion. I recently saw a report that said 90 per cent of all the things people worry about never happen. What a waste of energy! We have to train ourselves to take control of these emotions and direct that energy into positive thinking instead of putting up mental barriers like 'I could never do that because it is too hard,' or 'I can't because it is beyond my capabilities.'

Worrying is a waste of energy. Most of the things people worry about never happen.

Thinking back, I was probably a difficult person to work for when I had my signwriting business because my expectations were a lot higher than those of most people. I had the attitude that if I could do so many things without legs, then it should have been a piece of cake for my able-bodied employees. I hate to hear people making lame excuses for not being able to do things, or else blaming someone else for their shortcomings. I really don't like that at all. If one of my staff claimed they couldn't climb a ladder, for instance, I'd go out and stick the ladder up against the wall and climb up it myself just to prove my point. If you take the words 'no' and 'can't' out of your vocabulary all of a sudden life starts to look a whole lot different.

Goal-winning attitudes

Attitude is something you can't buy and it is what makes some people achieve their goals and others fail. That attitude determines whether or not you have the willpower to succeed. Take marathon runners for example. I've taken part in wheelchair marathons and I know what it is like to get to the 40-kilometre mark and then hit the wall. Your body feels like it wants to die. It doesn't matter how good or how fit you are there's always the mental as well as the physical challenge you have to contend with in competitive sport. Whether you're running in a full marathon or a half marathon or whatever, there comes a point where your body just doesn't want to carry you another step but you've still got another 2 kilometres to go. When that happens it is your strength of mind and willpower that are going to decide whether or not you finish the race. Some people never make it. They hit the wall and give up. That's the choice they make at the time. They may regret that choice at a later stage and think to themselves, 'Gosh, I could have done that last 2 kilometres if I'd pushed myself a bit harder.' But at the time their will to succeed just wasn't strong enough.

It is like anything in life; you can train for years and be incredibly fit and able, but somewhere along the line you're going to hit the wall and that's when self-doubt will creep in. You'll start asking yourself, 'Can I go any further?' or 'Can I really achieve my goal?' and 'Is it really worth all this pain and effort?' But I'll tell you what. That pain only lasts for a second, or maybe three or five, and then it is gone. Ask any athlete. And if you have the willpower to keep going, before you know it you've gone across the finish line and all those fleeting negative feelings are replaced with elation, exhilaration and euphoria because you've achieved your goal. Sure the pain comes flooding back into your body as you collapse on the ground from exhaustion, but you'll probably go through it all again another day because the sense of achievement is worth all the effort and anguish.

It is like childbirth. When a woman has a baby she endures all those terrible labour pains and vows, 'Never again.' But it is not long before she's dreaming about giving the newborn babe a little brother or sister! The pain becomes a dim memory and inconsequential compared with the reward that comes with it.

A positive attitude is the difference between achieving and not achieving goals.

Elaine and I rarely argue but if we do have a disagreement it is always very short-lived. Neither of us believes in bearing a grudge. We both have definite opinions about things so we do sometimes have different points of view and sometimes I try my hardest to make her see things the way I see them and, sure, I get a little frustrated when she won't. We may even get to the point where we argue about it but the argument never lasts long — 10 minutes at the most — because all of a sudden it is dealt with and we move on. So many people don't know how to deal with baggage. They don't know how to sit down and work an issue through and get a result. I believe that most of the time in everything I do I get a result whether it be for better or worse, and once I've done it I move on.

That's not to say that I've never made mistakes, but I feel that I have generally learnt from them. You can't be right all the time and you can't be a winner every time. But just because you're not a winner doesn't mean you're a loser. So many people don't realise that. As long as you've been prepared to give something a go and in doing so you've done your best then you've been successful.

Being successful is simply doing the best that you can. That's all the world asks of you.

Success is measured in so many different ways, and it is all a matter of what levels we set ourselves. I really believe that if someone truly wants to become a millionaire and they try hard enough then they'll achieve that goal. But, in saying that, for goodness sake don't sit around waiting to win Lotto. The reality is you have to work hard to make dreams come true.

You don't have to be a multimillionaire or an executive officer or a gold-medal winner. Society is always going to need ditch-diggers and dustmen, painters and plumbers.

I know many tradespeople who are very successful because they've built up a reputation for giving good service for money and they charge appropriately. As a customer I don't mind paying that little bit extra if I know I'm getting a quality job in return. That's how I ran my signwriting business. I prided myself on having a reputation for giving my clients exactly what they needed even if it wasn't always what they'd asked for in the first place! As far as I was concerned the reason people came to me was because I was the professional and they wanted professional advice and service. So if they wanted something I knew wouldn't work, I didn't believe in grovelling and saying, 'Oh well, if that's what you want that's fine by me,' and then turning out something I knew would be no good. I just couldn't do that and I had enough confidence and self belief to tell my clients. My reputation was at stake and I wanted to do the best that I could for each client. Not just because it was going to make me more money I hasten to add, but because I knew that was what they really needed and that in the long run it would therefore benefit them financially as well. More often than not, had I just done what the customer wanted it would have either been a terrible job or I'd have been out of pocket because I'd quoted them $5000 and then found the job cost me $10,000.

When I conduct workshops I stress the fact that business is all about people rather than products. It is about building relationships with your staff and your clients. That's what determines the success of your business and a lot of businesspeople lose sight of that. I always say that in business there are two types of people: the hunters and the farmers. The hunters are out there for a quick sale. They want their 10 bucks now. The farmers, on the other hand, are looking for the $500 they're going to get over the next 5 years and that's the important thing. They're thinking long term and cultivating those relationships with their clients. It is not about the 10 bucks you're going to get off a customer now but the $100 or the $1000 you're going to get off them over a period of time that's the important thing in business.

Another myth is that you have to live in a big city in order to make it big.

I went down to the southern most part of the South Island of New Zealand on a speaking engagement recently and discovered they have a tremendous shortage of tradespeople down there.

With the right attitude and determination you can achieve your goals anywhere.

Now the South Island may not be the warmest place to live in the middle of winter but the people are friendly, the scenery's magnificent and there's a shortage of workers in just about every trade — bricklayers, painters, concrete layers, truck drivers, farm hands — you name it and the South Island desperately needs it. Why? Because of 'The Great Drain North'. People are told that Auckland is the happening place; that in order to be successful you have to live in a big city like Auckland. But one third of New Zealand's population already lives there and as a result there are already thousands of unemployed in the city. Those who have a job have trouble getting to and from work every day because of the clogged motorways and poor public transport. Down south the air is cleaner, there's less crime and houses are cheaper. People could go to a place like Gore or Invercargill and get a job and become very successful but they're just not prepared to make the sacrifice. They've got the wrong perception of what you have to do to be successful and for some reason they think it is necessary to join the masses in Auckland in order to achieve their goals.

Invercargill's mayor, Tim Shadbolt, had the right idea. Originally in the concreting business in Auckland, he was Mayor of Waitemata for a term before losing his seat, and a few years later he decided to move south. Way down to the bottom of the South Island in fact. Now he's enjoying his third term as Mayor of Invercargill and a much more laid-back and fulfilling, not to mention cheaper, lifestyle. Radio and television personality Marcus Lush is another who has recently opted for what he calls a 'better quality of life' in the deep south, and of course our very own internationally renowned singer Suzanne Prentice has always lived in Invercargill. She frequently tours New Zealand and performs overseas but the rest of the time she just enjoys being a wife and mother in the southern city where she was brought up.

You can achieve your goals anywhere. I've lived in little old Tauranga all my life and I love it. It is a relaxed lifestyle with none of the hustle and bustle of the bigger cities but that hasn't stopped me from setting and achieving so many goals. I've found that the harder you strive the more opportunities seem to come your way. It doesn't matter where you live.

Colin Meads is another example. He's lived in the farming community of Te Kuiti most of his life and yet is one of the world's best-known rugby players. If he were an All Black today he'd be making heaps of money but he says he has no regrets about missing out on professional rugby:

'My brother Stan and I played in an era when it was a very amateur game but we made great friends and friendships and, of course, we had the major tours in those days. We'd go away for four months on a tour of the UK, for example, and they were fascinating times. These days if the All Blacks go away for a month they think it is a huge tour. And they just play test matches whereas we used to play a lot of provincial games. We'd have 30 or more games on a tour but these days when the All Blacks go

away they just play three or four tests. I've heard it said that the money aspect puts more pressure on players today but I think it was tougher for us because we had to hold down a job as well. We had to work for a living as well as play rugby and it was a hectic existence because we did a lot of our own training as well, whereas now they all have fitness trainers and it is a different world altogether.

'I certainly don't envy today's young All Blacks. We had some great times back in the sixties and we often talk about them when we get together for reunions. I've just been in Wellington for a Rugby Foundation function and I met up with some great old friends down there. And a couple of weeks ago I attended a reunion of the King Country-Wanganui team that beat the Lions in 1966. We all like to think we were a lot harder in those days because we had to work as well, and of course, back then you weren't allowed replacements during a game like you are nowadays.

'I don't have any regrets at all. As Tony says, I think it is important to enjoy life. I achieved all the goals I set myself as a player and then I decided I wanted to be an administrator. I tried coaching for a while but I wasn't very successful at it. You've got to realise your limitations in life and so I aimed to be a manager of teams instead and I achieved that. These days I'm just on the board of the King Country Rugby Union but I still follow the club and go down to the clubrooms on a Saturday. And I'll be over in Aussie later in the year for the World Cup. I've been asked to speak at several functions associated with the event. I probably average three or four speaking engagements a week but I never, ever get tired of talking about rugby.'

Besides his farming, rugby and business commitments, Colin has also been associated with the Intellectually Handicapped Children's

Society for many years. In fact he is patron of the society's Calf Scheme whereby farmers rear more than 5000 calves annually to sell on behalf of IHC, raising in excess of $1 million every year. And since his wife, Verna, had cancer several years ago he's also helped with several fundraising events for the Cancer Society. As if all of that's not enough, Colin is also a member of the Rugby Foundation that provides help for players who suffer serious spinal injuries while playing the game.

No doubt Colin is often asked how he finds the time to do all that he does. I know I am. It is as if we must have more hours in our day than other people, as if people think we have 30 hours in our day and that because they've got only 24 they've been short-changed.

> *We've all got the same amount of hours; it is what we do with them that counts.*

Remember the saying, 'Why put off till tomorrow what you can do today?' If you do choose to procrastinate that's fine, but don't blame other people for forging ahead of you up the ladder of success, for taking that opportunity that you had yesterday and doing something with it today. So you've been made redundant and now you're unemployed. You're certainly not going to get another job by just sitting around feeling sorry for yourself. There are umpteen steps you can take to give yourself the best opportunity for getting another job. First and foremost you've got to know what it is you want to do. Think about what you want to do with the next 10 years of your life. Perhaps you don't have any skills in the direction you'd like to take. So what? Enrol on a course and re-train. Once you've made up your mind what you want to do then you've got to get out there and try to find the job you want. It doesn't matter whether you pick up the phone or go door knocking as long as you do something constructive towards achieving your goal. Many of the most successful people in the world today are door knockers. And if the first 20 firms you approach don't want you, so what? You just keep knocking and eventually someone somewhere is going to take you on.

My wife Elaine used to be head chef at Cobb and Co. in Tauranga and she kept a list of all those people who turned up at her door looking for work. Whenever a vacancy arose she would always offer the job to the person at the top of that list. She never had to advertise for staff in the newspaper. It was so much easier to just pick up the phone and contact someone from her list, knowing that they'd been keen enough to come door knocking in search of work.

Some people say they can't give up smoking. Rubbish. You can do anything if you're determined enough. But you've got to want to do it. Whatever your problem in life, be it a weakness or an illness or a work or family-related issue, you *can* make it better for yourself because *you* are in control of your own life. And if you don't do something about it chances are no one else is going to, because most other people are too busy dealing with their own issues in life to worry about yours. No matter how much you love your family and friends and no matter how much they love and care about you, at the end of the day you do things for yourself because it is *your* life. Don't waste it.

Whatever your problem, you can resolve it because you are in control of your own life.

One of the things I'm getting better at doing is parting with possessions, possibly because we've moved house so many times in recent years. I look at an object and ask myself, 'Am I going to use this?' My new criteria is that if I haven't used it in the past 12 months then I'm never going to use it and so out it goes. Our new home is looking much less cluttered as a result. I think our lives are the same as our cupboards. They too can become cluttered with too much junk.

A friend recently moved out of the house he'd occupied for the past 16 years. You wouldn't believe how much junk he'd accumulated because he and his wife never threw anything away. He had to move because his wife had left him and he ended up having a nervous breakdown. He'd got to the point where his life, like his house, was full and he couldn't close the door. Everything was piling up on him and spilling out and he just couldn't handle it any more. So he had a nervous breakdown. How many people do you know who've got so much negative stuff running around in their heads they just don't know how to open the door, so to speak, and clean it all out? Elaine and I learnt so much from our friend about what a person goes through when they have a nervous breakdown, when their life falls down around them. We both have a much better awareness of what really challenges some people and hopefully we'll be able to ensure that we never have to go down that road. Because you learn from other people. That's why it is important to me to share my story with other people in the hope that they can learn from some of my experiences and make more positive decisions.

There are many accident and car-crash victims being saved today who years ago would have died from their injuries. They're living longer but with some horrific challenges in their lives. Like me, though, they've still got that precious gift of life. Like me, they've been given a second chance. And like me, they've got the choice of either taking that second chance and running with it, or wasting it by wallowing in self-pity.

It is not just those people with challenges in their life that I'm trying to reach, though. It is the so-called 'able-bodied' ones as well. Next time you see someone in a wheelchair don't walk past hurriedly, looking the other way. Give them a smile and a friendly greeting. Remember the saying, 'There but for the grace of God go I.' Just because they're amputees, or paralysed or suffer from cerebral palsy doesn't mean they're intellectually impaired or have no feelings.

It is important to hear other people's stories and share our own. I hope people can learn from my experiences and make more positive decisions.

Look at the famous British physicist and author Professor Stephen Hawking. He's had motor neurone disease for more than 30 years, which in itself is amazing because most people who have it don't survive more than 5 years. He's confined to a wheelchair and only able to communicate with the aid of a computer-generated voice and yet he's still regarded as having one of the finest minds on the planet. We can't judge a person by how they look. It is their attitude to life that's most important.

Looking on the bright side

Cancer seems to be so much more prevalent in our society these days, and sadly so many children seem to be suffering from it. I never fail to be impressed by those children I meet or see on television. More often than not their courage shines through like a beacon and their attitude towards their health and their future is so positive. Many of them have such special gifts and talents and it seems such a waste that they aren't able to pursue their dreams and realise their aims and ambitions in life. But they never seem angry or sad or bitter. I think we could all learn a lot from those brave kids.

We all need courage to persevere and the ability to laugh at our fears.

Life can be a pretty tough, mean place at times and you often hear people voicing their fears about things. Perhaps as a result of my accident things don't scare me any more. I laugh at fear. I think it is sad that so many people in the world take life too seriously and don't know how to laugh at themselves. Life is full of emotions; you've got to cry a little and laugh a little. But don't be afraid, and never harbour regrets. What's the point of dwelling on things that have happened in the past? You can't change them and the only person you're going to hurt by feeling sorry for yourself is you.

Life is full of ups and downs and you can go from hero to zero and back many times. Get rid of that negative thought or emotion because you can't change it so you might as well just let it go. It is history. It is just a story in the past and it is what you've learnt from it that's going to make a difference in your life.

It is so much more constructive to concentrate on the positives in life rather than dwell on the negatives. It not only makes you a happier and more fulfilled person but such an attitude is bound to have a positive spin-off on those around you as well. Not only will your family and friends enjoy your company more but your boss is also going to be grateful you're not carrying a chip around on your shoulder.

I believe that if anything else bad should happen in my life I now have the ability to deal with it. I've learnt from my mistakes and I've gained inspiration from other people. I haven't a clue what life holds for me tomorrow or next week or in 10 years' time. All I know is that I'll be able to enjoy the great things that happen, but by the same token I'm certainly not going to let the bad things ruin my life. Sure, every so often I get frustrated and think life sucks not having legs, mainly when I can't reach something on a shelf or in a cupboard. And there are a couple of things in motorsport, for example, that I'd really like to do but in reality they're impractical. I'd like to be able to race an endurance car with some able-bodied friends of mine but we'd have to have the car fitted out with hand controls, which would be a fairly costly exercise and it is just not that high on my list of priorities at the moment.

Often when I'm invited to address a conference I hear other speakers coming out with clichés such as 'Success breeds success,' and 'You're only going to get out of life what you put into it,' and, you know, all those inspirational sayings are true. All you have to do is sit and think about them and understand them and believe them. It is part of developing a positive attitude. That's why I karate-chop three boards at the end of my presentation — to make people sit up and think: 'If he can achieve so much in his life then so can I.'

> *It is not what happens to you, it is what you do about it that makes the difference. Concentrating on the positives makes you happier and more fulfilled.*

Many people, though, feel the risks are too great, but they aren't if you learn to mange them, which, among other things, is what I want to talk about in the next chapter.

The power of positive thinking

~ We only have one thought at a time and the choice is ours whether it's a positive thought or a negative one.

~ Bad, sad and negative things can be overcome. Don't harbour negative emotions. Put the bad times behind you and move on.

~ It is your attitude that counts. Everyone has negative baggage, but dealing with it positively is what counts.

~ Don't worry but instead direct your energy into positive thoughts. Most of the things people worry about never happen.

~ The difference between achieving goals or not is a positive attitude.

~ Being successful is simply doing the best that you can.

~ With the right attitude and determination you can achieve your goals anywhere.

~ We've all got the same amount of hours; it is what we do with them that is important.

~ We all need courage to persevere and the ability to laugh at our fears.

the risk factor | 6

> The big thing about risks is how you manage them.

One of the things that deters people from pursuing their dreams is the risk factor. They're too scared to give something a go because of the perceived dangers involved, be they financial, emotional, physical — or just the risk of the unknown. What they don't realise is that they're taking all sorts of risks every day of their lives without even giving them a second thought. For instance, every time you drive your car on the road you're taking a risk but it is one you just take for granted. All around the world people are being killed in road accidents every day but it is a risk we're all prepared to take and so we don't even think about it.

When you consider how many people do die in road accidents or from lung cancer or are injured in mishaps in and around the home — burns, electric shocks, falls, cuts and so on — it is a wonder we have the courage to get out of bed in the morning, let alone leave the house!

Risks deter people from pursuing their dreams, but we take numerous risks every day without even giving them a second thought.

On the other hand, throughout history there have been people prepared to take enormous risks in pursuit of their goals or to further their causes or follow their dreams. Explorers such as Vasco de Gama, Christopher Columbus and Captain Cook for instance. They all ventured into uncharted territory, not knowing if and when they'd see their homes and families again. At sea for months at a time, they lived in cramped conditions, having to contend with a lack of fresh food and the dangers of disease, hostile natives, mutiny among their own crews and, of course, stormy seas.

The sea has always held a fascination for humans, whether they're sailing on it, swimming in it or diving under it. As a child, I always admired Jacques Cousteau and I loved watching his TV documentaries. I'm in awe of all the risks he took throughout his years of underwater exploration. But they never deterred him because he was doing something he was passionate about and in the process he opened up a whole new world for millions of other people.

More recently New Zealand's Sir Peter Blake was following in Cousteau's footsteps in an effort to make people more aware of the need to protect life in, on and around the sea. After sailing in many gruelling races around the world in which risk taking was an everyday part of life it seemed as if he was opting for a slightly quieter lifestyle when he formed blakexpeditions three years ago. But Sir Peter knew better. Apparently he'd always been very much aware of the danger of modern-day pirates out there on the high seas and, sadly, on his second voyage up the Amazon River in South America in late 2001, he was shot dead when a band of gun-toting youths boarded his boat *Seamaster*. Sir Peter died defending his boat and his crew. Not just New Zealand but the whole world mourned the senseless killing of such a great man. But what a great legacy he left behind. He'd put this country's name on the world map of yachting not just by his achievements in the Round the World races but also by leading New Zealand to victory in the America's Cup in 1995 and again 5 years later. And 2 years after his death blakexpeditions continues its environmental mission on board *Seamaster*. Although his life was cut so tragically short, he had already achieved so much and made every second of his life count for something. He knew the risks and he died doing something he was passionate about and his name and memory will live on in our history books. Surely that has to be better than dying of old age after a lifetime of boredom or bitterness or regret over lost opportunities?

As the missionary and doctor Albert Schweitzer once said: 'The tragedy of life is not that we die, but what dies in a man while he lives.'

Another New Zealander who has inspired others around the globe is Sir Edmund Hillary. It is 50 years since he and Sherpa Tenzing conquered the highest mountain in the world, Mt Everest, and several jubilee celebrations were held in 2003 to mark the event.

> *The great explorers and adventurers were never deterred by risks because they were doing something they were passionate about.*

Since that first ascent just days before the Queen's coronation in June 1953, many hundreds of climbers have followed in Hillary and Tenzing's footsteps and many have also died in the process. Fifty years ago the risks involved for Sir Edmund and his team must have been enormous but he was pursuing a dream and all dreams have their risks. That's what makes fulfilling them so rewarding: the fact that you've overcome all the dangers and obstacles along the way.

As I write this it is only a matter of weeks since the space shuttle *Columbia* disintegrated as it re-entered Earth's atmosphere, killing the seven crew members on board. The disaster struck after what had seemed a near-perfect two-week-long mission in space. The crew's families were all watching television monitors and waiting for *Columbia* to land safely; their shock and grief was relayed around the world and onto our own television screens that evening. All those involved in the space programme are aware of the risks, however. There have been similar disasters before and no doubt there'll be more to come. Space travel is still very new and dangerous. As the brother of one of *Columbia*'s female crew members, Laurel Clark, noted: 'I'm just so glad she got to space and to see it because that had been a dream for a long time. When she saw the path to be an astronaut was open she went at it full throttle.' That's how we should all pursue our dreams — at full throttle. Like Sir Peter Blake, Laurel Clark died doing something she was passionate about. Some people take major risks and live to tell the story and, sadly, others die in the process. To quote Emerson: 'Neither you nor the world knows what you can do until you have tried.'

All dreams have their risks, but that's what makes fulfilling them so rewarding: the fact that you've overcome all the dangers and obstacles along the way.

A lot of the pursuits I indulge in, such as motor racing and flying, carry an element of risk. I have a bit of a need for speed and nothing is ever risk-free but I always take all the necessary precautions so that the likelihood of something bad happening is greatly reduced. Even then, disaster can strike when you least expect it.

I have an acquaintance who was riding his motorcycle out in the bush where I've been riding with my friends for years. I've fallen off my bike dozens of times without hurting myself too badly, and I'm sure this guy had as well. But one day he came off and broke his neck and now he's a quadriplegic. He'd taken the same risk so many times before but in that one moment on that one day his life was changed forever. There's currently a road safety campaign around New Zealand with big signs on the road asking, 'What's Around the Corner?' and the same question applies to our lives. We never know what life has in store for us so we should get out there and enjoy it while we can.

We should pursue our dreams at full throttle.

It is not always life that is at stake, of course. Businesspeople and entrepreneurs take financial risks and quite often win and lose their fortunes several times in a lifetime. Performers risk their reputation every time they go on stage or make a movie. Will the critics give them bouquets or brickbats? Sports teams run the same risk. Will they win or will they lose? Here in New Zealand sports fans have high expectations of their heroes, be they All Blacks, Warriors or members of our America's Cup team, Team New Zealand. We all knew Dean Barker and his team ran the risk of losing to the Swiss yacht *Alinghi* every time they went out on Auckland's Waitemata Harbour during their defence of the America's Cup. What we hadn't realised were all the other risks involved, such as the boom breaking and the mast snapping in half the way it did!

But who would have thought that a small, landlocked European country like Switzerland could have accomplished such a feat as winning the America's Cup? Indeed, many of his fellow countrymen thought Alinghi Syndicate head Ernesto Bertarelli was mad when he first came up with the idea. But for him it had long been a dream and he's living proof that dreams can and do come true. When he arrived back in Geneva with his jubilant team and the prized trophy he thanked them all for 'helping to make this incredible endeavour more than I ever dreamed possible.' Along the way he took many risks involving money, business, family and physical challenges but he stuck with his dream and now he's a very happy man.

While Bertarelli's key sailors, New Zealanders Russell Coutts and Brad Butterworth, no doubt feel as if all their dreams have come true, there's another Kiwi who's trying hard to make his life-long yachting dream a reality as well. As a child, Graham Dalton was so inspired by Englishman Sir Francis Chichester sailing solo around the world in *Gipsy Moth IV* that he vowed he too would accomplish that feat one day. It was a goal he never lost sight of and in 2002 he finally set sail from New York as a competitor in the Around Alone yacht race, an event that's been described as the ultimate ocean race and the greatest mental and physical challenge in any sport. Elaine and I saw all the boats taking part in the single-handed event when they had a month-long stopover in Tauranga at the end of the third stage. Unfortunately, during the next leg Dalton had to withdraw from the race when his 60-foot yacht, *Hexagon*, was dismasted off the coast of South America.

Obviously, he was very disappointed but he still hasn't lost sight of his dream of single-handedly circumnavigating the globe. In a newsletter on the Internet he said:

> *I know in my heart I will do this one day, but it will not be part of the Around Alone race. I have always said that you are successful in life not because of your successes, but because of your failures and how you deal with them. This still holds true, more than ever now. I won't give up on my dream.*

In an earlier release the solo sailor said:

> *You are your own greatest competitor and if you can face that challenge with honesty and dedication, success will come naturally. I don't believe in mediocrity; I do believe in setting goals, attaining them, and looking forward to the next challenge.*

If you think about it achieving goals is a bit like sailing. The going isn't always easy and straightforward and there is always the odd rogue wave to knock you off course when you least expect it. Sometimes you've got to tack back and forth a bit to dodge the difficulties, but if you stick with it and don't give up then your success is all the sweeter.

Sailor Grant Dalton has taken great risks to succeed, and is always looking to the next challenge.

We can't all be major risk takers like Ernesto Bertarelli, Russell Coutts or Graham Dalton, but from the minute we get up in the morning there are so many things we do in both our personal and business lives that involve some element of risk taking. I read that 10 years ago the average person had seven major, potentially life-altering decisions to make every day of their lives, be it driving a car, crossing the road or whatever. Today that figure has doubled to 20. That's how fast the world is changing. Many of them are unconscious risks, some are calculated and others are more extreme and unpredictable.

Managing risks

The big thing about risks is how you manage them. When I had my signwriting business some clients always wanted me to take the risk. But my attitude was: why should I? They wanted the job done; why should I carry all the risk? Why should I pay all the bills for materials and labour and so on and carry the customer's account until the job was finished and then hope they'd pay in full? Because there's never a guarantee that you're going to get paid. So I always requested that customers pay 50 per cent of the bill up front. Not many businesses do that but I did and it was very successful. In fact, some clients would pay me in full before the job was even started! On the whole, though, 50 per cent was a really good margin to work with because that way I didn't have to carry all the risk in the event of non-payment.

Life is all about managing the risks. We take risks every day but we can always have some level of control over them.

When you drive down the road you take a risk but you've got some control over that by how you go about it, whether or not you observe the speed limit and other traffic regulations, what conditions you drive in, and whether you are tired, stressed or intoxicated. As a pedestrian just crossing the road can be a risk as I found out in the United States recently, where of course the cars drive on the opposite side of the road to here in New Zealand. I'd just survived climbing Mt Kilimanjaro and had only been home a week when I had to fly to Miami for a speaking engagement there. I went to cross the road at a pedestrian crossing and forgot about the road rules being different. So although I looked both ways twice, I was actually looking in the wrong direction as I started to zoom across in my wheelchair and very nearly got skittled! I couldn't believe I'd just managed to climb the highest mountain in Africa with barely a scratch to show for it only to nearly get run over a week later! Which just goes to prove my point: we take risks every day of our lives without even realising it. Sometimes the little, unrecognised risks can be more dangerous and life-threatening than the big ones.

When you send your kids to school you're taking a risk by having someone else's perceptions of life instilled into them. The teacher's beliefs may well be very different to your own. But how many people actually go and quiz the teachers about their beliefs before sending their children to school? Not very many. As a parent does it matter to you whether your child's teacher was for or against the United States' war with Iraq? Does it matter if they're giving your child a different slant on events than you would prefer? Does it matter if the teacher thinks marijuana should be legalised and you feel equally strongly against such a move? Or that they favour corporal punishment and you don't? Whether it matters or not it is a risk most of us are prepared to take.

The thing about risks is that you can't sit around worrying about what might happen or what other people might think. Most of the things we worry about never happen, so why waste all that time and energy worrying? More and more people are being forced to take risks these days because of the way the world is changing. Many are being made redundant and having to re-skill in their fifties. They've probably still got 10 or 15 years of working life ahead of them and so they're having to seek new goals and pursue new dreams. Or perhaps they decide to take the bull by the horns and go after dreams they considered too elusive in their younger days. Look how many women are having babies later in life because they've become so career-minded that they only choose to start a family when they realise their 'biological clock' is ticking away. People are living longer and so need something fulfilling to do in their retirement; many are taking the opportunity to get the academic qualifications they missed out on in their younger days. It is amazing how many middle-aged people are going back to university or studying exciting new subjects at night school or seeking to keep up with the twenty-first century and become computer literate. Whereas it was always young people who had their 'big OE' (overseas experience) before settling down to a job and marriage, these days a lot of older people are opting to travel rather than stay home and play bowls or bridge.

Joy Bennett is a Bay of Plenty teacher and grandmother in her sixties who decided three years ago, just when most people are thinking of retiring, to go to India to teach at an international Christian school high up in the Himalayan foothills. Her late father had spent time there on a building project 20 years before and she'd always wanted to see the results of his labours and get to know some of the people he'd talked about. He was a well-known and much-loved character and is remembered fondly by many in India today. The trip there was daunting enough in itself. She flew to New Delhi and then had a hair-raising, eight-hour taxi ride north to a town called Musoorie, where the Woodstock School was founded more than a century ago. What a culture shock awaited her there! She had to boil all the water she used, even for cleaning her teeth, to avoid getting dysentery. Wild monkeys roamed the mountainside and were easily provoked into attacking, as were packs of wild dogs, and she had to keep her legs covered at all times to keep the leeches at bay! The mountain paths around the school were steep and narrow; she had to be careful not to get too close to the edge, especially at night. But Joy stuck it out, and once she got over her initial homesickness she grew to love the place. She became especially attached to her pupils and decided to stay on for another two years.

Many older people are taking the risk of study, travel or new work — and enjoying the rewards.

Sadly, while home on leave, she discovered she had cancer and spent the next six months undergoing surgery, chemotherapy and radiation treatment. But Joy has indomitable faith and courage and as

I write this not only has she just been given a clean bill of health by her specialist, but she's getting ready to return to India for another three years! She's a truly remarkable woman and she's experienced so much at a time when most people are looking for a much quieter life. Sure, she's taken risks and faced some gruelling challenges in the past few years, but her life is so much the richer for having done so. Although she'd be the first to admit she misses her family and home comforts when in India, this time when she returns to Woodstock she won't be on her own. Her eldest daughter and son-in-law have chosen to follow in Joy and her father's footsteps and have signed a four-year contract to work at the school. In fact they're already over there and loving it.

Health problems are one of the biggest challenges people have to face these days. Not just cancer, like Joy had, but so many other debilitating if not deadly diseases and viruses, which can strike anyone at any time. Who would have thought that cheeky young actor in the television comedy *Spin City*, Michael J. Fox, would have been diagnosed with Parkinson's at such a tender age? It used to be considered an old person's affliction, but not any more. New Zealand's Olympic runner John Walker also has the disease. What a cruel fate for one who used to thrill the world with his record-breaking feats on the track? Walker and Fox both admit they've been through the agonising, 'Oh no, why me?' reaction to their plight and now they've moved on and are making the most of their lives. Both are actively involved in helping other sufferers to understand and manage their condition better.

We can't sit around wondering when the next disaster is going to strike.

Sure, we all suffer knocks in life, but you've just got to bounce back up and take the good with the bad. Today's world is full of new challenges and opportunities and we are so lucky to have such a huge choice. Life is so exciting. Don't waste a minute of it. Think of something you'd really like to do and go out there and do it. If there's something you really want to do, whether it is an adrenalin-pumping adventure-type activity or a quieter, home-based hobby, don't let anything or anyone stop you. It is your life and your choice — go for it. That first step towards a goal can often seem like a giant one into the unknown but once you've summoned up the courage and determination you'll realise it wasn't that hard after all and you'll wonder why it took you so long to take it.

Embracing new opportunities

As you get older your goals tend to change for one reason or another. It has been my experience that the more I achieve the more doors of opportunity open for me and therefore the greater the choice available. But if you're in a wheelchair like me, you still have the odd battle with bureaucracy to contend with. After I had qualified to be a pilot, I was still over the moon about the achievement and could quickly see many possibilities opening up for me. One of my goals was to circumnavigate New Zealand solo in an aeroplane and perhaps even become the first disabled pilot to cross the Tasman Sea solo. It would have been another first for the history books and another feather in my cap. Since then, however, I've hit a few snags with Civil Aviation and I've decided that rather than waste my life arguing with the authorities I'd rather move on and conquer other horizons. I have proved I can fly a plane and that was the main challenge. The problem is that in order to keep flying I need to clock up a certain quota of hours, which is not easy if you're busy, and I have to have a special medical each year, at a cost of $400, just so someone can confirm what I already know — that I don't have any legs! It seems to me that Civil Aviation want everyone to be a perfect specimen living in a perfect world in order to fly aeroplanes these days. They call it a privilege to be able to fly an aeroplane, whereas I actually think it is a right. It seems to me there's always someone out there trying to make another rule to stop you from doing what you want to do.

Rather than get stressed out about it, however, I'm just focusing on things I can achieve without having to battle bureaucracy in the process. Like scuba diving, for instance. I've always been fascinated by what lies under the sea. Jacques Cousteau was always a hero of mine because of his achievements, especially the fact that he invented the aqualung and then used it to experience a totally new world. There is so much to see. Some underwater explorers find something phenomenal like 20 different species of fish every time they dive.

The more I achieve the more opportunities appear and the greater the choice available.

I'm not into pillaging the seas like a lot of people who go out and get their crayfish, scallops, snapper and so on every weekend. Sure I enjoy a spot of fishing occasionally, but I also enjoy seeing fish alive and swimming under the water. I've been snorkelling in the Great Barrier Reef and seen massive clams that are nearly a metre across with lips of magnificent colours — purples, reds, yellows, greens and magentas. Since I became a professional speaker I've travelled to engagements in all sorts of exotic locations, but until now I've always had to content myself with just snorkelling. It wasn't that I didn't want to dive deeper. I just wasn't allowed to. Once again I was the victim of red tape and people's perceptions. Although there are always plenty of dive boats at these places the diving instructors are not allowed to take 'disabled' people down. They've decided we have more difficulties and more challenges than supposedly able-bodied people when it comes to diving, but that's not necessarily true. The main difficulty I've noticed is that if you have a physical disability your buoyancy tends to be different. But this is easily overcome by adjusting your weights. Because I don't have legs for counterbalance and to give me the necessary leverage I hang weight belts off my shoulders as well as around my waist to keep me horizontal. I've had some little pockets made up to wear on my arms so in future when I go overseas I'll just take them with me.

To get my diving certificate I did a four-week course that involved about 10 hours of classroom work and four open-water dives of a minimum of 20 minutes each. You have to perform skills under water, such as filling your mask up and then clearing it, and taking your regulator out, retrieving it and putting it back in. If you run out of air underwater you have to share air with another diver. You have to practise all those sorts of skills you might need to use in a real-life diving situation.

I did the course with a group of others who were physically challenged in some way and our instructor was an experienced PWD (Person With Disability) instructor. Interestingly, he had difficulty getting his fellow instructors to help with our course, presumably because they were afraid of our perceived disabilities. However, a group of guys who were doing the professional divers' course came along on one of our dive days and our instructor got a letter from one of them a few weeks later. A middle-aged Maori guy who was going for his professional divers' certificate wrote to say it was the best dive experience he'd ever had. He said he'd really enjoyed being there with the PWD divers and it had given him such a great sense of fulfilment. He'd probably never had that sort of contact with disabled people before and, unfortunately, there are all too many others like him.

Apart from the buoyancy challenge, I've also discovered that people who've lost limbs or had operations on their spines tend to get a build-up of nitrogen in their bloodstream when they dive. The pressure that builds up underwater can cause nitrogen to gather in a particular area of injury, such as where you've had a limb amputated or a spinal operation. That can cause nitrogen narcosis or deep nitrogen sickness when you return to the surface. But you can overcome the problem by not surfacing too quickly, by staying at 5 metres for three minutes to allow your body to equalise.

Since getting my certificate I've been out several times as a buddy to other guys who've been doing their first open-water dive off Karewa Island in the Bay of Plenty. We go down to about 16 metres and it is absolutely fantastic. I don't find it a disadvantage at all not having legs or not being able to wear flippers. I propel myself with my arms in a breaststroke sort of style and I can keep up with the guys using flippers because diving is usually a casual type of activity, not a race. It is all about being able to take the time to look around and appreciate what's under the sea. Those giant clams I mentioned before are usually about 3 or 4 metres under the water and in the past I've been able to sort of duck dive down to that depth with a snorkel but of course I can't stay down there very long like that. It is going to be great now to be able to put an aqualung on and dive down to around 5 to 10 metres and explore some of the spectacular coral reefs around the world. In future when I'm invited to speak somewhere that's noted for its great diving I'll try and spend an extra day or two there so that I can see some of the underwater sights. I've had several speaking engagements on Hamilton Island off Australia's Queensland Coast and in future when I go there I'll definitely be taking my wetsuit, weights and mask with me. As a recreational diver I'm only allowed to go down to a depth of 30 metres but I'm quite happy to stick to that. Wrecks are usually found much deeper but we've got the old tug *Taioma* outside Tauranga Harbour so I can always explore that if I want to. We also have our very own volcano, White Island, off the Bay of Plenty coastline and I've heard the marine life around that has to be seen to be believed.

Meeting challenges with confidence

I guess I'm lucky to be married to someone who understands my need to be always trying new things and pushing the boundaries. People think Elaine must worry herself sick about me but on the whole she knows my capabilities and trusts me not to make mistakes. I must confess, though, that I've ended up in hospital a couple of times after mishaps while motor racing. But there are times when she does get anxious and I know she wasn't too keen on the idea of me climbing Mt Kilimanjaro:

'One of the questions I'm most often asked is "Don't you worry about him?" Well, of course I do, especially when he's racing motor cars or motor bikes and doing things like that but, on the whole, because we've been together 25 years, I've got used to it. I know he has to do these things to satisfy his need for speed and so that's fine. But the hardest part about Kilimanjaro was the fact that I didn't know what was happening most of the time he was away. We normally keep in touch all the time; either I'm there with him or he calls me as soon as he's finished whatever he's doing. But for 12 days while he was climbing Mt Kilimanjaro we couldn't communicate at all. The television crew had a satellite phone I was supposed to be able to call Tony on but one of them lost it before they even started the climb! I'd heard so many negative things about Africa before he went there, about the danger of bandits for instance. Apparently they'll kill you for just 10 dollars and I knew the documentary team was taking over a million American dollars' worth of equipment with it, so that really frightened me for a start. Then there was the fact that the mountain itself kills several people a year, although of course thousands of people make their way to the summit every year, and live to tell the story! To make matters worse for me, it was the first time we'd spent Christmas apart for 25 years, and I'd so looked forward to having the festive season all together in our new home with our children and two grandsons. And then, even after they'd climbed the mountain, Tony wasn't allowed to come home for New Year because the crew wanted to do more filming in Kenya. So it was a very worrying time for me but Tony's a survivor and I should have known he'd be alright.'

My track record in wheelchair mountaineering wouldn't have filled Elaine with confidence. Before I went to Africa I hadn't done any, except that as a teenager I was pretty nifty at getting up and down

Mt Maunganui — on my backside! I'd be with a group of my best mates, such as Porky McGill and Ivan Shannon, and we'd grab a few cans of beer and head up to the summit of 'The Mount' as lots of young guys did back then, and probably still do today. Trouble was, it would take me about three and a half hours to get to the top and by the time I got there the others had usually drunk all the beer. I was faster going down, though. I used to slide down the steep side on my bum. It was a bit rough and rocky in places but I always made sure I was wearing at least three pairs of pants for protection! Those were the good old days and adventures like that were quite exciting. More recently, about a couple of months before I went to Africa, I took my grandson Houston to Mt Ruapehu to see the snow and we climbed right to the top of a pretty steep slope. I didn't think I was going to be able to make it, to be honest, but we dug a track as we went and I'd shove my bum into a foothold and then push down hard with my stump and drag myself up. It took me about an hour to get to the top but young Houston and I were both pretty pleased with ourselves when we finally got there.

Elaine has had enough confidence in me to encourage me to give everything a go, and fortunately that confidence has been rewarded.

When you're taking risks of any kind you have to think of the repercussions for your nearest and dearest as well as yourself. I was mad about cars and motor racing and speed when I first met Elaine so she's always been used to that aspect of my life and I guess over the years she has come to trust my judgement and know that I don't take unnecessary risks. I must admit I was a bit worried myself about how I was going to get on in Africa. Even my self belief was put to the test at the thought of such a daunting exercise, especially when I learned that up to 10 people a year die on Kilimanjaro, usually from altitude sickness, exhaustion or a fall. Sure there were all sorts of risks involved. Altitude sickness is the biggest killer but there's also the risk of dehydration, hypothermia or getting a stomach bug thanks to the rather unsanitary conditions up there, especially as we stayed on the mountain twice as long as most other climbers. But there's nearly always something you can do to lessen the risks or at least manage them. Look at me — I'm still alive so I must have done something right. I took plenty of warm clothing for a start, and wet-weather gear. I had special plastic pants made and I also bought several pairs of leather gloves. I took pills and drank lots of water to combat altitude sickness and Elaine packed me some emergency rations for which I was very grateful. But I was amazed at how ill-prepared many of the people were that I saw on Mt Kilmanjaro. I saw people going up there in hiking shorts and T-shirts with just light packs on their backs. They didn't manage the risk at all because the weather on the mountain can change in minutes. I guess it is the same here in New Zealand when people go into the bush or out in boats ill-prepared. But the best risk-management decision I made was to take a companion with me so that I had someone I could talk to in English and who would be moral support if I had to stand up to the demands of the director and his colleagues. I rang my friend Peter Hillary, Sir Edmund's mountaineering son, who put me onto a guy called Matt Comeski. Matt was a seasoned climber who also happened to be a student nurse in Auckland. What's more, he was dead keen to go with me so I couldn't have found a better buddy for the expedition.

> *There's nearly always something you can do to lessen the risks or at least manage them.*

But you know, sometimes the risks aren't half as bad as you expect or as people, and especially the media, lead you to believe. I knew before I left for Africa that I'd be spending several days in Kenya after the climb, but I didn't dare tell Elaine because I knew she'd get alarmed. We're always hearing about the political unrest in that country and about riots and bombings and so on and indeed a bomb went off in a hotel in Mombasa less than a month before we were there. I was in Nairobi over Christmas and New

Year, during a general election. We were warned to stay in our hotel because there were going to be riots and demonstrations but I have to report that I didn't see a single sign of trouble. However, if I'd told Elaine I was going there she'd immediately have considered it a dangerous place to visit and would have been even more worried about me than she already was. She was much happier once she knew Matt was going with me as my 'advocate', as she called him. As for me, having made history by becoming the first disabled person in New Zealand to learn to fly solo, I was keen to see if I could become the first person in New Zealand — if not the world — to get to the top of the highest mountain in Africa in a wheelchair. The next two chapters give an account of my attempt to do just that.

The risk factor

~ Don't let risks deter you from pursuing your dreams.

~ The great explorers and adventurers were never put off by the risks involved because they were doing something they were passionate about.

~ All dreams have their risks, but that's what makes fulfilling them so rewarding: the fact that you've overcome all the dangers and obstacles along the way.

~ You should pursue your dreams at full throttle. You can't worry about what people think or when the next disaster is going to strike.

~ Life is all about managing the risks. We take risks every day but we can always have some level of control over them.

~ The more you achieve the more opportunities will appear.

~ It is your life and your choice — embrace new opportunities and challenges with confidence and self belief.

off to africa 7

It is my belief you can change your whole life simply by changing your attitude.

One thing about being busy is you don't have time to worry about what lies ahead, and in the weeks before my trip to Africa, boy, was I busy! I did manage to get some trips to the pool for some serious swimming, which is great exercise for the arms and upper body, and I went on a crash diet in order to lose a bit of flab. But really I'm pretty fit anyway because I'm using my arms all the time either to push my wheelchair or to propel myself around when I'm on my bum.

Elaine and I also did a bit of research on the Internet to learn more about Mt Kilimanjaro and what sort of conditions I could expect. We tried to concentrate on the positive aspects. We had been hoping to see the video the Korean television crew had taken on their advance trip but it didn't arrive till after I'd left, which is probably just as well because Elaine saw it later and was shocked at how difficult the climb looked.

Anyway, just when I might well have started feeling nervous and having second thoughts I was commissioned to do a week-long road show throughout New Zealand for an insurance company. It started in Auckland and went right down the North Island and then on to Christchurch and Dunedin. I was addressing mostly self-employed insurance brokers and had to give the same talk in a different town or city every day. No sooner had I finished the road show than I flew to Perth to deliver a speech there. That was two days before I was due to embark on the African expedition. That whole period towards the end of November 2002 remains just a blur but at least life was never dull. It was a bit hard on Elaine, though, who was left to handle a lot of the last-minute arrangements and of course, do all the worrying for both of us!

So I flew back to Auckland from my Perth engagement on 29 November, which also happened to be the day I was due to fly out to Korea. Elaine met me at the airport and we shot into town to see our son Luke. Then there was just time for a change of clothes and a bite to eat and back we went to the airport to meet my 'minder', Matt Comesky. Luke and his girlfriend, Shannon, came along to farewell us and I was very grateful they were there because by this time Elaine was pretty upset about the whole thing and it was really hard leaving her when she was so distressed. I'm flying around the world all the time for speaking engagements and that doesn't bother her, but this was something very different. It was the unknown element that worried her. I was more concerned about her than I was about myself. I felt pretty confident that I'd be able to handle whatever lay ahead, especially having Matt with me.

Matt hadn't climbed Kilimanjaro before but he had done K2 twice, which is pretty impressive. At 8611 metres (28,250 feet) K2 is the second highest mountain in the world. Mt Everest is 8848 metres (29,028 feet), which is only 237 metres (778 feet) higher than K2 and some climbers maintain K2 is a much more difficult challenge than Everest. Matt reckons it is a very daunting climb. But whereas Everest and K2 are scaled by very experienced climbers who mount highly organised expeditions to get to the top, Kilimanjaro is a much more commercial proposition. You just plan your own trip and when you turn up at the foot of the mountain there are guides to lead you up to the summit via a series of huts. New Zealand's Prime Minister, Helen Clark, and her husband Dr Peter Davis, climbed Kilimanjaro in January 1999, the same year she was elected to run the country. They'd lived to tell the story and hopefully so would I!

It was a pretty long flight to Korea so it was good to have Matt to talk to and share a few laughs with. When we touched down at Inchon International Airport we had to wait two hours for the documentary director to pick us up. He'd been given the wrong time for our arrival. When he finally arrived the director/producer turned out to be Joung Hoe, or Jeanie as we preferred to call him — otherwise known as 'Mr One More Time' — the same guy who'd produced the first Korean documentary I was in. We found it easier to call him Jeanie because so many people in Korea are named Joung or Kim or Lee or Hoe, and it can get very confusing at times. Jeanie took us to our hotel in Seoul, where we rested for an hour or so before being taken to meet the clothing manufacturer who was supplying our clothes for the climb. As requested Elaine and I had sent my measurements over a few weeks before because of course I'm a lot bigger in the body than most Koreans, who tend to be short and slim. But as I'd found before, the Koreans seem to operate on the spur of the moment. So I was introduced to Mr Kim, the owner of Sierra Torro, a well-known alpine clothing company and one of the sponsors of the documentary, and he took one look at me, his jaw dropped and he said in his broken English: 'Oh. *Wery* big!' Then he looked across at Jeanie and back to me and repeated soulfully: 'Oh, wery, *WERY* big.' It was at that moment I realised he didn't have any clothes to fit me and that it was just as well I'd thought to bring some sub-zero stuff with me from New Zealand. I have no idea what happened to the measurements we'd sent but they measured me again and said they'd try and get some clothes made ready to send with a couple of members of the film crew who were travelling to Tanzania a week or two after us. We were going to be filming various segments of the documentary before we got to Kilimanjaro so we didn't need the entire crew straight away.

The rest of our day in Seoul was spent doing newspaper and television interviews and I got to meet the other two 'stars' of the show. Soo Young was a young blind woman in her mid-thirties and Hong Bin was a well-known Korean climber, or alpinist as they call them over there, who'd lost all his fingers on both hands to frostbite. He'd been climbing in Canada some eight years before and got caught in a very bad snowstorm. He'd lost his gloves and couldn't get down and I guess he was lucky to be alive, but obviously it hadn't put him off climbing. Apparently he'd climbed Kilimanjaro before he lost his fingers so he knew quite a bit about it and the conditions we were likely to expect. We also met Soo Young's helper, Kyung Mi, and the camera director, Mr Kim, who was in charge of filming. They had this big flash NZ$150,000 camera — a huge thing — as well as a smaller video camera in case anything happened to the big one, which it did. More on that later!

Within about 12 hours of arriving in Korea we were on our way back to the airport to catch the plane to Tanzania. I couldn't believe the size of Seoul. It is a massive city and I've never seen so many cars in my life. I was pretty pleased to get out of it quite frankly. Twelve of us met up at the airport, including two alpinists provided by the Korean Highway Corporation. The Corporation, which looks after all the Korean motorways, sponsors an alpine team and so they sent two of its members along to help with the documentary. Their names were Hun Park and Me Gong. They were really good guys and very experienced climbers, although neither of them had been up Kilimanjaro before. So 12 of us flew out that night and we were later joined by two other film crew members plus forty porters.

We flew out of Seoul straight for Osaka in Japan, which is more or less in the opposite direction to Tanzania. Don't ask me why. I still don't know but it certainly wasn't for lack of asking. It is part of my culture to choose the quickest route and get to where we're going as fast as we can. But the Koreans were quite happy to just sit there and accept the situation. I don't know whether they had a sponsorship deal with a specific airline or what the story was. So while Matt and I got all agitated about going such a long way round to get to Africa, the rest of the team weren't the slightest bit interested or perturbed. They just accepted it and I knew at that point that things were going to be a little bit difficult at times. But when I thought about it later it occurred to me that sometimes you have to go in the opposite direction in order to find the right path to where you want to go.

I can remember the late Sir Peter Blake once saying that sometimes, when he'd been sailing around the world, he'd had to go hundreds of miles in the opposite direction because that was the way the wind was blowing. But he always knew that eventually the wind was going to change and he'd be able to sail back on course again. He didn't know when that would happen but he knew for sure that it would. I think it is the same with life. Sometimes things don't go exactly the way we've planned them and we're always going to be faced with challenges — the wind's going to be blowing in the wrong direction. But if you don't lose focus of where you need to be, the boat will still get you there. It is so easy to just stay focused and carry on and that's something I learnt on the plane. As a Kiwi I don't like wasting time. I want to get going. But my way is not the only way. In other countries people are quite happy to go 'round and round the houses', so to speak. They still actually reach the same goal but they have a different way of going about it. That night on the plane all the Koreans in our party just sat there and didn't give a damn where they were going. They could have been going via Osaka or Timbuktu for all they cared but they knew that eventually they would end up in Tanzania. So we flew for two hours to Osaka, where we had an hour on the ground, followed by an 11-hour flight to Dubai, with another two hours on the ground there, and then six hours to Nairobi, Kenya, and another two to get to Dar es Salaam in Tanzania. We seemed to be in the air for a heck of a long time and of course this was on top of our flight from New Zealand to Korea, so it was a long time since we'd had any decent sleep.

When we finally got to Dar es Salaam it was only to find the paperwork hadn't been filed properly. The film crew had hired a Korean travel organiser living in Nairobi to make all their travel arrangements. He was another Mr Kim, not to be confused with Mr Kim the camera director or Mr Kim the alpine clothing manufacturer. It seemed that the Koreans wouldn't deal with the Tanzanians for fear of being ripped off. As it turned out they'd probably have been far better off hiring locals to do the job, but that wasn't our choice to make and so Matt and I decided fairly early on that we would just go with the flow and whatever happened happened.

Suffice to say there were a lot of challenges ahead of us long before we even got to Kilimanjaro. One of them was usually being the last to know what we'd be doing the following day. That was very frustrating and whether it was due to lack of communication or the language barrier I don't know. But we'd wake up in the morning and find everyone else had had breakfast and was waiting to get on the bus and we'd only just got up because no one had bothered to tell us the itinerary the night before. It was inevitable that things would come to a head at some stage, and as far as I was concerned the sooner it happened the better.

After waiting two and a half hours at the airport at Dar es Salaam for Mr Kim the travel agent to come up with the right documentation we finally boarded a bus bound for our hotel. Well, wow! If there was a five-star hotel in Dar es Salaam ours wasn't it. In fact I'd go so far as to say that ours was a *minus* five-star hotel. I'd never seen anything like it in my life! To get to it we drove down these pot-holed back streets lined with tumble-down tin shacks. It was just unbelievable. I kept reminding myself that I was in another country to shoot a documentary and that things weren't always going to be how I expected them or what I was used to. (It turned out there was a five-star hotel in Dar es Salaam, but we couldn't stay there because the Koreans hadn't pre-booked our accommodation and the place had been booked out by a United Nations conference.) So we got to our minus five-star hotel and of course there weren't any ground-floor rooms and there wasn't a lift and so it was out of my wheelchair and up the stairs on my backside. And because the restaurant was on the first floor that meant we had to keep going up yet another flight of stairs with some of the other guys having to heave my wheelchair up behind me.

It was when we got to the dark little alleyway on the second floor that we discovered Matt and I, who hardly knew each other at that stage, were expected to share not just a room but the bed as well! That was when we started to lay down the law about our expectations. We explained that while people from other cultures might be quite comfortable sharing a bed with a semi-stranger it wasn't our way and that in fact it was totally unacceptable as far as we were concerned. So Matt got a room across the alleyway and I got a supposedly first-class room. I'd hate to have seen what the budget rooms were like! The carpets were absolutely full of fleas for a start and because I don't have legs I was always wondering what I was sitting on so I made sure I wore my plastic pants and a pair of gloves wherever I went. I was grateful, though, that the room was air-conditioned, because it was very hot over there and when you left your room the heat would hit you like a brick wall.

From my window I looked down on lots of little tin huts and one day it rained and I was amazed to see all the women rush out with buckets and bowls to catch the fresh water as it poured off the roofs. Apparently they use it for washing and cleaning. Even after it has been boiled they say it is still not advisable to drink it. Fortunately, the film crew always supplied us with plenty of bottled water. In fact, the bottled water in Tanzania has the brand name 'Kilimanjaro' so we drank a lot of that. Only trouble was, the local beer had the same name so you can imagine the confusion every time we went to a hotel and ordered a Kilimanjaro! If you didn't specify whether you wanted a beer or a water you'd be bound to get the wrong one. Swahili is the language of Tanzania, although a lot of Africans speak very good English. We had picked up an interpreter in Dar es Salaam, a great guy called Georgie.

He'd spent five years with the Tanzanian Army in North Korea so he was very fluent in Korean and also spoke very good English as well as several other languages. He was fairly well known locally as an interpreter and a 'Mr Fix-It' and he stayed with us throughout the trip. He was forever getting the team out of trouble. Mainly trouble, I might add, that Mr Kim the travel agent had got us into in the first place! Besides Georgie we were also joined by another good guy in Dar es Salaam, our bus driver, Winston.

We were in Dar es Salaam for three days and most of that time was spent waiting to get permits and other paperwork sorted out. As with Seoul I just couldn't believe the number of people and cars in the city. A far cry from little old Tauranga, my home town back in New Zealand, that's for sure. One place we did go to was the city of Bagamoya, 70 kilometres north of Dar es Salaam and just off the coast of the island of Zanzibar. It was a two-hour drive to get there and we were an hour and a half late starting out because for some reason Georgie was late turning up. It reminded me a bit of Fiji: 'No Hurry, No Worry'. I also noted in my diary:

I now know where all the vehicles from around the world come to die. Elaine always thought it was Vanuatu but she's wrong. It is Tanzania! Both the vehicles and the roads are in a shocking state and everywhere you go there are people on the side of the road repairing diffs and gearboxes. There's no such thing as a warrant of fitness here.

Bagamoya and Zanzibar were the last places in Africa to abolish the slave trade, and there's a slave museum there so the crew decided to get some footage of Soo Young, Hong Bin and me walking around it. They were eager to include some African elements in the documentary. Our museum guide, Peter, got a real shock working with Korean TV, especially when our 'One More Time' friend got going! At one stage we were driving along a stretch of beach to where the slaves where shipped over to Arabia. It was an awesome setting, a real old fishing village.

Anyway, our bus got stuck in the sand and so I jumped out and walked about 500 metres on my hands and backside the way I usually do. I get along very fast like that and when I turned round to see where the others had got to they were all just standing there with their mouths wide open. Some of them thought I'd fallen out of the bus and when they realised I was merely powering along under my own steam they couldn't believe their eyes. Jeanie thought it looked so good he decided to make me do it 'one more time' again — and again — until I'd spent about an hour going backwards and forwards in the blazing sun. Then when they got the bus out it was only to discover it had a flat tyre and so there was more waiting around.

Late that afternoon, when we'd finished filming in Bagamoya, we set off across the Masai Steppe for Arusha, which was a 10-hour bus trip. In fact, we weren't supposed to be travelling at night because the roads are rife with bandits after dark but we went anyway. Georgie always had his gun at the ready and I had every faith in his ability to handle any situation. That's not to say I wasn't just a trifle scared at times, especially when we got to the first checkpoint and Georgie began loading his gun! We had to go through five checkpoints on the way and at each checkpoint all the guys had guns and there were spikes over the road. But Georgie seemed to know everyone and he buttered them up by calling them all 'Commander', which made them feel important and then he'd slip them 5000 shillings (about US$5) and they'd be as happy as heck and off we'd go. It was coming up to Christmas and they all wanted to fill their Christmas fund so everyone was backhanding like crazy. Georgie said they'd stop a truck and the driver would pass over his logbook along with 20,000 shillings (US$20) and they'd let him through. But if the driver didn't do that then the guards would go through the truck looking for contraband because the black-market trade is rife. Even if they didn't find anything they'd smash a light and then fine the driver 50,000 shillings (US$50) for having a broken light. And the poor guy wasn't allowed back on the road until he'd paid it. So it was easier just to slip them a backhander at every checkpoint.

Halfway to Arusha, in the middle of the night, we ran out of diesel so we had to get some from a group of black-market guys on the side of the road. I'd been a bit apprehensive about Georgie's gun to start with but at that hour of the night it was comforting to know he had it, although he reckoned he'd probably never have to use it. He said that although the bandits had a habit of holding up vehicles and stealing from the passengers, they tended not to kill people because they'd invariably be tracked down and killed in turn by the police and the army. Not only that, their families would also be made to pay to serve as a lesson to others. Everything's a life or death situation. If someone's caught poaching in one of the parks they're shot on sight. The guards know that's what they have to do. So, given all these facts, I not surprisingly stayed awake all night until we got to Arusha, unlike my Korean friends who had an unbelievable knack of falling asleep the minute a bus or plane started moving forwards. You'd look back and there were all these heads lolling back with mouths wide open. As soon as the bus stopped for a fuel or toilet break they all woke up and got off the bus and walked around, and then the minute it took off again they'd all fall asleep before the driver was even out of second gear. It was unbelievable how they did it.

I had almost as much fun watching them as I did looking out of the window. Not that I could see much in the dark. The roads were long and straight and on either side were people walking along with buckets of water on their heads. Why they were doing that at night I don't know and how the driver managed not to hit any of them I don't know either because it was pitch black outside.

We finally got to our hotel in Arusha at 1.30 a.m. It was another minus five-star wonder but at least I only had to climb up one flight of stairs this time. I desperately needed a good sleep but was awoken at 6.00 a.m. by the loud sounds of car horns and people yelling. Another day had begun. The hotel manager was from Moshi, at the foot of Kilimanjaro, and he'd climbed the mountain many times. He'd also known an American in a wheelchair who'd tried to reach the top but had been unable to make it. However, he reckoned we were far better prepared and felt the fact that I could get out of my chair would help a lot. He was sure we could do it so that was encouraging. That morning the crew filmed us browsing around the Arusha markets and then we were told we were moving to a lodge in one of the national safari parks. Jeanie warned us it was not good accommodation, which said a lot considering the minus five-star hotel we were vacating! It was about this time I started counting the days until I could fly home to my lovely, clean, comfortable house. Little did I know what lay ahead!

It turned out that for the next three days we were to be filming in a Masai village. The Masai people are a nomadic tribe whose whole life revolves around their cattle, sheep and goats. The animals provide milk and meat for the tribe as well as skins for clothing and bedding. And they also provide one other vital commodity as I found out to my horror. Dung! Every morning the young Masai take the animals out onto the steppe to graze for the day but at night they're brought back into the compound to sleep among the huts, so not surprisingly the whole place is covered in dung. At least 4 inches deep! The smell is unbelievable and there are flies absolutely everywhere. I had never seen so many flies in all my life. The children had flies under their eyes and in their ears and up their noses. I was forever waving my hand over the kids' heads trying to flick them away but they'd just go from one child to the next. I had a strong insect repellent on my arms so they didn't come near me at first but the minute the Masai people turned up the flies would descend in clouds. I soon found out why. We were welcomed into the village by a Masai elder, who in a gesture of goodwill gave me his brightly coloured robes to wear. It was then I realised why the flies were hanging round. Boy did they smell. They were absolutely putrid and I had to wear them every day for the documentary! As soon as I got dressed up in them the flies descended on me from all directions despite my insect repellent.

It was a huge cultural shock, and I know I'm judging them by the way I live my life, but who's to say their way is wrong and mine is right? Everyone talks about being luckier or more fortunate than others but most of those people probably considered themselves wealthy compared to some other tribes in Africa. They were certainly very friendly and welcoming and it was a marvellous experience to spend time with them.

The film crew had negotiated a fee with the Masai and come to an arrangement about what we would be filming. They wanted to show Hong Bin, Soo Young and myself participating in village life. Now the little huts in the village were made of twigs and — believe it or not — cow dung! So every morning after the young people had taken the animals out for the day the Masai women would get big aluminium bowls and fill them with dung, which they would then smear like cement all over the outside and the inside of the little houses. A sort of repairs and maintenance procedure. The cow manure is spread all over the walls and left to harden and crack. Can you imagine the stench? So guess which activity the film crew chose for us to take part in first? You've got it! To our horror we were each given a bowl full of dung and told to start slapping it onto one of the huts. I thought Matt had gone along to protect my interests and take care of my health but I have to say that all he did was just stand there and roar his head off. Oh, and take heaps of photographs to show Elaine when we got home. Thanks a bunch, Matt. Of course, he didn't have to take part in the ritual because he wasn't part of the documentary and when I looked questioningly at him — no, make that pleadingly — he just laughed and gave me the thumbs up. In the end the only way we could cope with the experience was by seeing the funny side and we ended up having a lot of laughs.

Because Soo Young is blind, Hong Bin and I were holding her hand as she scooped up fists full of dung and she was squealing her head off. And because Jeanie insisted on filming us from every conceivable angle we spent at least two hours up to our elbows in the smelly stuff. No doubt the sequence will be so short when it goes to air that viewers will miss it if they blink. Needless to say, I couldn't wait to get back to our lodge that evening so I could have a shower but when we got there it was only to discover it had no power. Nice one, Mr Kim. Our friendly travel organiser had struck again! Fortunately, we found a camping ground not too far away with bungalows that weren't too bad and I finally got my shower and then we all viewed the day's film footage amid much laughter before having dinner and going to bed.

I might add that during this time it wasn't just the Masai culture Matt and I were learning about. We were also getting to know a lot about our Korean friends and in particular their passion for chicken and rice (or maybe it was just that they felt this food travelled best). Every meal seemed to consist of the same thing and I must confess we both got a bit sick of it after a while — I was very grateful for the supplies Elaine had packed for me. We did go to a couple of nice restaurants in Arusha, though, especially a pizza place that was fantastic. Imagine that — eating an amazing pizza in the middle of Africa!

The next day we went back to the Masai village and we were driving along a track across the plains when Jeanie suddenly yelled out: 'Stop, stop, stop.' So the bus stopped and Mr Kim the director got out and after a while we all piled out and there was a cow lying on the ground about to give birth to a calf. But what had caught Jeanie's eye was the fact that a group of young kids aged about eight or ten years old were hitting the cow on the head with canes. There were three of them as I recall, all wrapped up in the brightly coloured garments the Masai wear, and apparently they were beating the cow about the head to prevent it from going into shock. Or perhaps the pain of being beaten around the head was supposed to take its mind off the pain of giving birth. I really wasn't too sure. Meanwhile another group of kids was tending a herd of goats nearby. Although the children all seemed to be looking after animals by themselves, there was usually a Masai elder sitting behind an ant mound or a bush somewhere watching over them and, sure enough, as soon as we started taking photographs a man appeared suddenly, protesting vehemently. You don't do things like that without first paying money to the Masai, so Georgie took the man to one side and negotiated a price while we watched the kids deliver the calf. It was an amazing experience. One boy continued to hit the cow on the head while another one grabbed the calf's feet and tried to pull it out. He was slipping and sliding all over the place and then another youngster reached in and pulled the calf's backside round and the next minute the wee thing shot out while we were trying to explain to Soo Young what was happening. Then one of these 10-year-olds grabbed the calf and dragged it round to the front of the cow who was heaving away and slowly regaining consciousness after being bashed on the head for half an hour! The mother started to sniff and lick its infant and at that point the kids began to kick and beat it again to make it stand up. Not surprisingly, it was a bit shaky, and so was the calf when they picked it up and tried to get it to stand. But as it got stronger and stopped wobbling all over the place and falling down, its instinct led it to the cow's udder and its first feed. The children's arms and legs and clothes were all covered in blood and slime and dung but it didn't worry them. I could have stayed there all day watching them and, as it turned out, when we finally reached the Masai village I rather wished I had!

By the time we got there it had started to rain and you can imagine what the compound was like once all that dung got wet. And you can imagine how thrilled I was having to wheel my wheelchair backwards and forwards through the mire of manure. Nevertheless we filmed a whole lot of sequences including Hong Bin, Soo Young and me helping a couple of the Masai women to prepare an *ugali* meal inside one of the huts. Ugali is like a stiff porridge and is probably their staple meal. So the two women got a pot of water boiling over the fire. But wait. Wasn't that the same pot they'd had cow dung in the previous day? Afraid so! They've got these aluminium pots they use for absolutely everything: for fetching water from a spring some distance from the village, for cooking — and for collecting dung! So there they were, boiling up the water and I'm looking at Matt and he's looking at me. He pointed out that at least it was boiled water. Thanks, Matt. So they tipped a packet of ugali in and kept stirring it until it turned into this thick porridge stuff and then they scooped some out with their fingers and offered it to me to eat. What could I do? I had to put it in my mouth and pretend to enjoy it: 'Oh yum, very good, very good.' I then turned my head and quietly spat it out, wiped my mouth on my already very smelly Masai wrap then beamed at everyone and added: 'That was lovely.' Meanwhile Matt, as usual, was having a great laugh at my expense.

We soon stopped laughing when they brought along a goat to kill in our honour, though. That was too much for me and I had to get out, but there was worse to come. The film crew had arranged for Hong Bin and me to take part in a special Masai ceremony that had something to do with proving one's manhood and involved drinking fresh cow's blood. They get this little wee arrow with a cup attached to it and stick it in a big vein in the cow's neck. The blood squirts into the cup and then they remove the arrow, stick a finger over the punctured vein, drink the blood and then refill the cup! By this stage I was squirming around in my wheelchair saying, 'Oh man, I don't want to do this, I do *not* want to do this.' In the end I was allowed to just pretend to drink it for the camera and then the cup was drained by someone braver than me, after which I was filmed proudly brandishing the empty vessel. Hong Bin drank it, though — he is a tough cookie — and he ate the ugali as well but being a woman Soo Young didn't have to do it. Apparently the Masai mix cow blood up with heaps of stuff including ugali. I tell you, even the chicken and rice tasted good that night.

Another rather disconcerting habit we came across at the village was the Masai men's habit of blowing their nose vigorously with their hand before shoving it forward to shake hands with you. Oh boy! My whole reason for coming to Tanzania was to climb Mt Kilimanjaro and I was desperate to remain as fit and healthy as possible for that but there were times when I thought I was going to be killed, quite literally, by kindness. Matt had thought his aim in life was to get me up the mountain and back in one piece. He hadn't bargained on all these other challenges to his nursing skills as well. But, hey, we survived and in terms of experience and understanding we're definitely the richer for it. Nevertheless, every time I got back on the bus I'd get out the packet of Dettol wipes Elaine had packed for me and I'd rub myself all over and I'd spend 10 minutes in the shower every night when we got back to the camping ground.

Given their living conditions and lack of hygiene it is small wonder that nothing and no one there dies of old age. Only one in five children survives to the age of five years old. Whereas in New Zealand attaining the age of five is an occasion of great excitement because that's when you start school and have so much to look forward to, it is seen more as a miracle among the Masai people. Because they're constantly on the move, going from one village to another to find grazing for their animals, they are rarely near a hospital. If they need urgent attention they have to travel miles to the nearest town so more often than not they just let nature take its course. Many of the older people get tuberculosis and it is small wonder they get damaged lungs because they keep a little fire going inside their huts 24 hours a day, seven days a week and the dung-lined walls and ceiling are black from the smoke.

The oldest Masai are probably only about 40 years old but they look 20 or 30 years older. The animals don't get to see old age either because they're killed either for their meat or skins. Having said that, they were very happy people, always laughing.

After filming with the Masai people for three days we returned to Arusha and the following day headed out to the world-famous Ngorongorongo National Park. We had to go in four-wheel-drive Jeeps and Landrovers and it took us four hours to get there because those vehicles aren't the fastest in the world. When we finally arrived at the main gates — surprise, surprise — we didn't have the proper papers and permits and we weren't allowed in. So we left a couple of the guys there to sort things out while the rest of us went to the nearest town where we found a minus three-star hotel and had chicken and rice for dinner before turning in for the night. Well, actually the others had chicken and rice for dinner. By then I'd reached saturation point as far as that particular gourmet delight was concerned and so I chose instead to stay in my room and settle for a couple of snack bars and a can of Diet Coke. Matt and I roomed together most of the time but Matt was really adventurous and was always off taking photographs and exploring so I enjoyed spending a bit of time to myself in my room.

Our instructions were to be up at five o'clock the next morning to be at the gates of the park by six. But when we got there, we discovered that Mr Kim the travel organiser had made another mistake and the gates didn't actually open until 7.00 a.m., which meant we had a whole hour to kill. So we had to just sit there and wait and eat bananas for breakfast. I must say, however, that when we eventually got into Ngorongorongo Park it was a fantastic place. It is 600 metres down in the crater of an extinct volcano between the Serengeti Plain and Lake Manyara, and the wildlife is amazing. There are something like 25,000 animals within the crater itself, including elephants, zebras, lions, black rhino and wildebeests.

You've probably seen documentaries about it on television. But I've discovered that you don't always get the right perception from watching television or reading the newspapers. For instance, you can sit down in your favourite armchair and watch a one-hour programme on the Ngorongoro Park and you'll probably get to see every large animal there is there. But it is not quite so easy when you actually visit the place because that one-hour programme you watched probably took at least a couple of months to film, whereas most visitors are only there for a day. We travelled down rough tracks and saw little gazelles running around. A bit further along we saw some big buffalo and then we drove past a waterhole where there were thousands of beautiful flamingoes. We began looking around for elephants but we soon discovered they were not that easy to find. We watched some hippopotamuses sinking under the water, leaving only their nostrils sticking out, and the park ranger found some lions for us, but still no elephants. At one place in the forest we came across great piles of elephant dung so the big animals couldn't have been too far away, but they were nowhere to be seen. We found a cheetah that had just killed a baby gazelle and was munching on it and, in the end, on our way back we were finally lucky enough to see a herd of elephants. It made me realise that you could in fact drive around that park for days and not see one of the huge beasts, so nothing is ever quite as it seems on television. Next time I see David Attenborough pick up a rock and excitedly find a very rare snake underneath it I won't be so impressed. I'll know it probably took his researchers weeks to find it and then put it there for him to 'discover' the minute the camera rolled.

Nevertheless, Ngorongorongo Park was an amazing place and the scenery was magnificent too. We did a lot of filming there and it was late at night by the time we got back to Arusha, where we spent another two days, mainly resting, before setting off for Moshi at the base of Kilimanjaro. On the way to Moshi we had to stop at Kilimanjaro International Airport to pick up the two extra members of the team who'd flown in from Korea via Amsterdam. They were Mr Chou, who was overall funding director for KBS Television, and Mr Lee who was the financial director and chairman of the Korean Highway Corporation, one of the sponsors of the expedition. I'd met Mr Chou in Korea and he was a really great guy and very amusing. Kilimanjaro Airport is designated international because it gets direct flights from Amsterdam. While we were there Jeanie decided to film Matt and me to make it look as if we'd also just flown in.

Then it was off to Moshi and as we drove along we got our first glimpse of Kilimanjaro. You can't usually see it during the day because it is obscured by cloud but first thing in the morning and last thing at night it is an awesome sight. Quite daunting too, but I kept looking at it and telling myself, 'It ain't that big really!' There are really only two types of attitude or thought: positive and negative. You can't have an in-between thought and I looked at the magnificent mountain that day with its glacial ice cap and air of mystery and I knew I would get to the top. I thought, 'This is what we came here for and this is what I'm going to do.'

So many people had told me before I left New Zealand that I was mad for even contemplating such a feat. In the end I came to the conclusion that they said these things because they would never ever dream of doing such a climb themselves and maybe they were afraid that I *would* do it. That I *would* succeed. Perhaps they didn't like to see me taking risks they weren't prepared to take themselves. Perhaps they were envious. Who knows? I've had people tell me I make them feel inadequate but that's certainly not my intention.

I think some people think it is all about one-upmanship, that I'm trying to prove that I'm better than somebody else. But it is not like that at all. I do the things I do because I want to, because I enjoy doing them and because I have the opportunities to do them. And if you choose to do something I believe you should give it the best you can and if it doesn't match up to someone else's level it doesn't matter. It is how you measure yourself that counts. If some people want to sit in the safety of their home all day that's their choice, but they shouldn't criticise those who want to tackle new challenges and achieve new goals. It is too easy to concentrate on the negative side of life. In fact, we're brought up in a negative world where bad news makes headlines. It is my belief, however, that you can change your whole life simply by changing your attitude.

That night after we'd reached Moshi, I talked to Elaine on the phone and was relieved to hear that everyone at home was okay. She said she'd seen the video the advance party of Koreans had made of Kilimanjaro and she thought it looked really hard going. But I got up the next morning at first light and went outside to see the mountain at its clearest and I still thought I could do it. I still had a positive attitude and I was determined to give it my best shot.

We spent a couple of days in Moshi making last-minute preparations for our climb. There were a lot of things to be organised and Georgie spent a lot of time tripping backwards and forwards with the Koreans, getting permits and so on. Matt and I spent the time adapting my wheelchair for its ascent. When I'd first agreed to take part in the climb I'd been promised a special climbing wheelchair that had been made in the United States but when they showed it to me in Korea it was obvious it wasn't going to be suitable. In fact the only thing that could remotely qualify it as a 'climbing wheelchair' was the fact that it had big, fat mountain-bike tyres on it. So we had to come up with an alternative and while we were in Moshi Matt and I and the Korean alpinists discussed ways of altering my own chair so that I could take that up the mountain. Because its front wheels were so small they would have dug into the mountainside and tipped the chair over so we had some big, long steel poles made that clamped around the chair like a rickshaw. The idea was that I would push on the main wheels with a porter fore and aft pulling and pushing on the poles whenever necessary.

Although we were in what could probably be called a Third World country it was surprising what we could get done in Moshi. We went to a little corner bike shop where a guy was working out of a tiny shed with rubbish everywhere but he did a great job. First, we changed the wheels over so that I had mountain-bike wheels on my chair to give it more stability. Then we went to an engineering company, where they got two lengths of pipe and welded bits onto them and made bolt clamps and fitted them onto my chair. Once it was finished I had to have a bit of practice to try and get used to the modifications before we started the climb. We also did some more filming. People at a nearby coffee plantation village gave us some food for the trip and so they were filmed presenting it to us. There were a lot of banana trees there with rotten leaves everywhere that absolutely stank. Elaine rang while we were in the middle of filming and they wouldn't let me take the call. She talked to Matt and said she'd ring back that night but she didn't so that worried me a bit. What made matters worse was that it wasn't until we got halfway up the mountain that Mr Chou, who had the only satellite cell phone, confessed that he couldn't find it anywhere and thought he must have left it in a restaurant back in Moshi! So not only did I not know how my loved ones were back home in New Zealand but Elaine had no way of keeping tabs on me either!

After leaving the coffee plantation, for some reason Jeanie insisted on filming us all crossing this wretched river. I still don't know what relevance it had to the documentary because there is no river on Kilimanjaro but Hong Bin and Soo Young had to wade through and there I was on my bum, up to my armpits in water and, boy, was it cold! I was wearing my plastic pants and they were great until the water got in over the top. It was quite a fast-flowing river too and there were a couple of big rocks we had to jump either over or around. When it goes to air in Korea the documentary will be 90 minutes long and I guess they want it to look as dramatic as possible. No doubt then I'll find out where the river slotted into the scheme of things. Anyway, after that bit of excitement it was back to our hotel to get changed and pack our bags and then it was back onto the bus. Kilimanjaro, here we come!

8 the crown of africa

Every day you move forward is a good day and you just enjoy the moment because you never know what the next day's going to hold.

We got to Marangu Gate at the base of the mountain and waited three quarters of an hour while the film crew haggled with the authorities over our permits. The crew wanted a permit for 10 days but the authorities only wanted to give them one for eight days. It is quite expensive to do the climb and of course they wanted more money for the two extra days. There were hundreds of porters there and two of them came up to me and introduced themselves as August and Godlizen. It turned out they were to be my own special porters and Matt and I both got on well with them straight away. All the gear was laid out on the ground and as the porters' names were called out they'd each come forward and pick up a bag. It was really well done. We had 40 porters accompanying us. One carried a generator for the power and another carried 20 litres of petrol for the generator. That was just to provide power for the cameras. Then there was everyone's clothing and food. It was a logistical nightmare but it all seemed to work out well. Our chief guide was a guy called Dismus and there was another one called Sylvester. They were both very nice people and very knowledgeable guides. Their mission was to get us to the top of the mountain.

We finally left the gate at about half past four in the afternoon, which is quite late to be setting out for the first hut, the Manara Hut, at 2744 metres (9000 feet). Fortunately, they got a four-wheel-drive vehicle to take me, Soo Young, Hong Bin and my two porters the first five kilometres up the track. Well, when I say fortunately perhaps I should qualify that. The Jeep was like something out of *Indiana Jones* and the driver was a real hard case. I know a lot about cars and I really didn't think the thing was going to make it. It was running on three cylinders and the driver was spraying ether in the carb to try to get it to go but to no avail. He had the bonnet up so I took a look under it and found a spark plug lead off. I put it back on and the engine spluttered a couple of times and away it went! Well, the driver hugged me as if he'd won the lottery. But we still had to get the Jeep up the track and that was another adventure. I thought the gearbox was going to fall out and the driver only used two gears — slow and slower. We finally got to the end of the road just on dusk at half past five and we still had 4 kilometres to go to the hut so we put my wheelchair together and off we went.

The first part of the track was up through rainforest country and it was really rough going over rocks, stones and branches. Luckily, my porters were very strong and once they knew I wasn't going to break we were away. The way we'd rigged up my chair like a rickshaw worked really well. I pushed forward on the rear wheels while one porter held the front wheels up and pulled a bit and the other guy gave us a push up the rough bits when we needed it. If the going got really tricky I'd just jump out of my chair and they'd drag it up while I went up on my backside till we got to an easier part and then I'd jump back in again. We hadn't gone very far before it got dark and Matt had to use his torch to guide us, but we reached the first camp safely at half past seven. The rest of the team had begun walking an hour before us so they'd all arrived ahead of us.

The huts were small A-frame buildings, each containing four bunks with a mattress and pillow on each. The porters brought us a bowl of hot water to wash in and some fruit and they heated up a can of baked beans for me, which I had with a cup of Milo. It tasted great. Then I was ready for bed. It had been a long and exhilarating day and I was really tired. As it turned out I wasn't to get a lot of sleep that night or in fact all the time I was on the mountain because the battery recharger on the mask I wore at night virtually gave up the ghost. I suffer from the fairly common sleeping disorder known as sleep apnoea, whereby I stop breathing several times during the night. It was a bit scary, especially as we got higher up the mountain and the air got so much thinner. Sometimes I'd get the mask to work for two or three hours but then I'd have to just lie there and hope that if I did drop off to sleep I'd wake up again in the morning! Trouble was, if I did manage to snore off, so to speak, then Matt and whoever else was sharing my sleeping accommodation would suffer because without my mask 'snore' is the operative word! I spent a lot of my spare time on 'Kili' trying to repair and rewire the recharger but my breather never seemed to work for more than three hours at a time.

The next day we were supposed to climb 12 kilometres from the Manara Hut to Horombo but because the crew did so much filming we only got halfway there and even that took us seven hours. The going was so much harder as well. I'd thought nothing could be tougher going than the previous night but I was wrong. The rocks and stones were so much bigger and I kept having to get out of my chair and walk a hundred metres or so on my backside. As we began to gain altitude I also found myself becoming breathless much more quickly. The filming was stop, go, stop, go all the time. Jeanie was up trees taking photographs one minute then running ahead and jumping out of bushes. Then half-way there Hong Bin started arguing with the directors, maintaining that he and I and Soo Young should be doing the climb all by ourselves without the help of porters! That would have been quite impossible as I quickly pointed out and everyone agreed with me, except Hong Bin of course. So after an hour of argument we decided we would carry on as before but let Hong Bin manage by himself. He is a strong guy both physically and mentally, and it took him quite a while to back down and let the porters help him again. Meanwhile, most of the porters had gone straight up to Horombo but because they knew we weren't going to make it that day they'd left us with all the stuff we needed for the night. So we found a campsite on the side of the mountain and pitched our tents between the rocks. The weather was lovely and sunny and warm and there was a fantastic sunset that night. It was just amazing because we were well above cloud level and when the clouds cleared we were looking down over the lights of Moshi and Arusha. We all had good sleeping bags so we had a comfortable night and the sunrise next morning was absolutely spectacular.

Actually, I tell a lie. I had a comfortable night but Matt wasn't quite so happy. We were supposed to be sharing a tent but I remember rolling over in the early hours of the morning and realising that I was alone; Matt wasn't lying there beside me. I peered around and noticed the tent flap was open so presumed he must have gone out for a pee. This was about 3.00 a.m. I lay there waiting for him to return and after 10 or 15 minutes had elapsed I began to get a bit worried. So I stuck my head out of the tent and bellowed loudly: 'Matt, Matt, where are you?' 'Over here, under a tree,' came the reply. 'What are you doing over there?' I asked, somewhat bemused. 'Trying to get some sleep,' came the rather tetchy reply. 'You're making too much noise you b...d!' Obviously, I'd been snoring again. I stared over at Matt under his tree for a few seconds, wondering what to do, and then I thought, 'Oh well, it is not that cold and if he wants to sleep outside so be it.' I clambered back into my sleeping bag and went back to sleep.

We were up by six o'clock and the porters brought us all breakfast and hot water for a wash. Then we packed up and set out for Horombo. We got there in about four or five hours, which was really good, especially as the crew was filming all the way and it was pretty steep in places. The porters who'd gone on to Horombo the night before came back to help us the next day. Those guys were just amazing the way they could walk up and down the mountain so effortlessly, especially considering all the gear they carried as well. The vegetation on this leg of the climb through the alpine meadows was fairly sparse because they had had fires on the mountain a few months earlier and all the plants and shrubs had been destroyed. Things were just starting to regenerate but the landscape was still black. We reached Horombo in the early afternoon and it was great to see all the huts there. Like seeing civilisation again! Well, almost. The boys found Matt, Jeanie, Georgie and me a hut and some hot water and then we all went into the main hut to see the day's footage on the monitor. It looked really good.

While we were there about 30 people stopped by on their way down the mountain. Of that number 23 had made it to the top, including a man of 76, so Mr Lee felt better as he was 57 and the oldest in our team. That night I was really exhausted and my arms were killing me so I went to bed early as we had another early start the next day.

There was actually a little breakfast hut at Horombo but the next morning my porters brought me breakfast in bed. How's that for service halfway up the highest mountain in Africa? Room service on Kilimanjaro! It was great and I really appreciated it. By this stage we were starting to get quite high — 3167 metres — and the next hut, Kibo Hut, was right at the base of the peak. It was another 1500 metres up and the going was very steep and rough so there was no way we were going to get there in one day. Instead, we headed for a place called Last Water, where we were to camp for the night. It was a gloriously clear morning with great views and although it was a bit steep at first the tracks weren't too bad. We kept stopping along the way to do some filming, and then disaster struck. Mr Kim the cameraman slipped and fell and dropped the big digital camera, damaging the lens.

We waited around for about an hour to see if they could fix it and then decided to carry on up to Last Water. Apart from the mishap to the camera it was a really happy day. Matt and I and our guys and another group of porters had a few laughs and we were all singing away and having great fun. We'd be meeting people coming back down the mountain and we'd all be calling out to each other: 'How're you doing?' I didn't meet any other New Zealanders up there but there were a lot of Germans, Austrians and Japanese. Probably only a third of them had made it to the top, though. I was a little bit worried that maybe I wasn't going to be able to make it after all but I'd decided to just take each day as it came and do the best I could. One of the things Matt said to me was that 'Every day you move forward is a good day and you just enjoy the moment because you never know what the next day's going to hold.' He was very encouraging. He told me not to have any expectations because the weather, the terrain and the mountain itself can take it all away from you in an instant. I thought about Kilimanjaro and the fact that it had been there for thousands of years and would still be there thousands of years after I'd left it so all I could do was take each step as it came and not have any preconceived ideas or expectations.

We got to Last Water, so named because it is the last water point on the mountain, at about one o'clock. There's no water at Kibo, the next hut; it has to be fetched from the stream at Last Water. Matt and I pitched our tent on one of the few little flat areas and just relaxed. Some of the team had headaches and stomach cramps but I was feeling really good. We had a meeting to discuss what was going to happen about the camera. Jeanie decided that everybody would have to go back down to Horombo while two of the crew went right back to civilisation to get the camera fixed. Now right from the very start I had made it clear that no way was I ever going to retrace my steps. I'd told them, 'I only move forwards; I don't go backwards and I'm not going back to Horombo.' I pointed out that they still had the smaller camera so they could still keep filming but they said it wasn't digital and it wasn't the same quality and I said I didn't really care. As far as I was concerned we'd come to climb the mountain and that was my major priority. In the end it was decided that Mr Chou and Mr Kim the organiser would take the camera lens away to get fixed while the rest of us would carry on and wait for them at Kibo Hut.

So the next day the two men set off back down the mountain to Moshi — goodness knows how long it took them — from where they caught a taxi for a 10-hour drive across the border to Nairobi in Kenya. Meanwhile we packed up camp and headed on up to Kibo Hut. It was a fresh, cold morning and the going was pretty steep out of Last Water but it flattened out a bit going across the saddle and everyone had a turn at the front of the chair. We had to have lots of stops because the air was getting pretty thin at 4500 metres and it was really cool when the sun disappeared. The landscape was the most barren I had ever seen and looking up towards the peak it seemed so steep I wondered how I was ever going to make it. We climbed 1000 metres that day and I had a lot of fun with the porters whenever we stopped, playing hand games such as 'knuckles and slaps'. The last kilometre was really hard going, steep with loose stones and by now, at 4700 metres, the air was getting really thin.

We all had big smiles on our faces when we finally reached the Kibo Hut and realised we were the first of our group to arrive. Next up the hill was Mi Gon carrying Soo Young, who had collapsed on the way up. I thought she must have just been exhausted but it turned out she had altitude sickness. Hong Bin was with them and he was also exhausted and had a powerful headache and was short of breath. Kibo comprised one big building with seven bunkrooms containing 12 bunks per room. The rooms were cold and damp and most people only stayed there between five and seven hours before leaving at one o'clock in the morning to make the final ascent. We ended up spending five nights there waiting for Mr Chou and Mr Kim to return with the camera.

After being carried up the final stretch to Kibo, Soo Young was taken inside the building and Matt was called in to help as she was in a pretty bad way. She was vomiting and Matt was really concerned about her and thought she might have to go back down to Horombo. However, after getting some fluids and Gastrolite into her she seemed a bit better, but by then just about everyone had bad headaches, including Matt. But not me! I couldn't believe I felt so well apart from feeling very homesick and nervous about what lay ahead. I didn't sleep much that night and I heard a group of people leave for the summit at about midnight and return five hours later, having not made it. The following day I saw many others who had got to the top but some of them were really tuckered out.

Next morning Matt and the other alpinists on the team headed up to the next campsite to check it out and then Matt and Mi Gon went on to climb Uhuru Peak or the so-called Crown of Africa — the summit of Mt Kilimanjaro. He was very tired when he got back and went straight to sleep. He said it was very hard going and that he'd thrown up on the way there. Nearly all the rest of the team had some form of altitude sickness. I just felt very bored. I hadn't packed any books or magazines because I didn't think I'd have time to read. And there was no way I could contact Elaine thanks to the mobile phone being lost. Reception was very patchy on the mountain anyway and at Kibo the only place you could use a phone was on top of a big rock about half a kilometre away from the hut. Fortunately, the porters had their own special phone and so the Koreans pitched a tent on top of the rock and sent two of the porters to sit up there and wait for phone calls from Mr Chou and Mr Kim in Kenya. Although I felt sorry for the two guys involved, it nevertheless struck me as very funny at the time. They had to sit up there in their tent on a rock in the snow and every time they got a phone call they'd clamber down and run all the way to the hut to tell Jeanie who'd then have to run all the way back to answer the call. So there were guys running backwards and forwards through the snow half the night. It all seemed a bit of a farce.

At last word came through that the lens was fixed and Mr Chou and Mr Kim would be rejoining us as soon as possible. After they'd done the

10-hour journey back from Nairobi to Moshi and then climbed back up the mountain, of course! What a circus.

In the meantime we had several meetings to try to decide what we should do about Soo Young. The only way to get over altitude sickness is to go back down to a lower level and so eventually Jeanie decided to take her back to Horombo and then bring her back up again the next evening. He was talking about getting a helicopter in to take us to the top but he had no clear plan of how or when and I was rapidly running out of patience. I told him that if he wasn't better organised by the next evening Matt and I and our porters would be on our way back down the mountain, documentary or no documentary. I wrote in my diary that I was so fed up at that particular point I would gladly have paid for Matt and me to fly back to New Zealand from Nairobi. However, I felt I had to give Jeanie one more chance to get his act together, mainly because so many others had invested time and money in the project. Matt had already reached the summit so he didn't mind one way or the other but we decided to stick it out another day. So Jeanie took Soo Young back down 1500 metres to the Horombo Hut on a one-wheeled stretcher, accompanied by Hong Bin who was also feeling sick, and we prepared to sit it out yet another day. Our original two-day stay at Kibo had turned into five days and all we could do was watch the other climbers come and go.

About 20 people a day went through the hut and word soon spread that we had a nurse in our midst. Matt had made a point of taking along everything that might be needed in an emergency, such as pills, fluids, drips and so on. So people would come staggering in out of the snow suffering altitude sickness or whatever and asking to see 'the doctor'. I thought it was a great joke and the minute I saw a prospective patient approaching I'd amuse myself by bellowing loudly for 'Matt the Medic'. People would come up to me and say, 'I understand you have a doctor with you' and Matt would get very embarrassed and say, 'I'm not a doctor, I'm just a student nurse.' Sometimes when he saw a group of climbers approaching the hut he'd quickly walk away and try to hide but more often than not he'd end up dispensing a couple of Disprin or whatever and telling his 'patients' to 'Call me in the morning if you need me.' We got a great kick out of Dr Matt's surgery on top of Kilimanjaro!

For my part, I spent most of the time in my sleeping bag because that was the warmest place. There was no heating in the hut and with its concrete floor everything was cold and damp. It was minus 14 degrees Celsius at night. We talk about experiencing four seasons in one day but up there you can get four seasons in just one hour. You can go from snow to brilliant sunshine to sleet and hail all within the space of an hour. One morning when it snowed quite heavily and the ground was covered in about 5 centimetres of the stuff we all went out and had great fun slipping and sliding all over the place and having snowball fights. But it soon melted and we were left with bare rocks again.

Most of the time, though, I just watched the other climbers coming and going from the hut. Because the climb's a commercial venture most people get up to Kibo in two days, arriving early in the day and then having a meal and a rest before leaving again at midnight to go to the summit. However, a lot who reached the hut while we were there would look up at the steep haul to the top and say, 'Oh no, I'm not going up there!' Those who did attempt the climb usually got to the summit between 7.00 and 8.00 a.m. and then they'd climb back down to Kibo, rest again and then go back down to Horombo. I couldn't sleep very well up there in the thin air, especially without my mask, so I'd just lie and listen to them setting off in the middle of the night. More often than not I'd hear some of them return within two or three hours either because the going was too tough or they just felt too sick. I was amazed at how many people got altitude sickness. They'd have violent headaches or be vomiting. I couldn't believe I didn't get it. I had a very slight headache one day but it wasn't bad. And that was all. Perhaps it was because I drank a lot of water. Matt and I had stockpiled some bottled water and every day I drank 2–3 litres and yet I never needed to go to the loo because I got so dehydrated up there. Water comes out of your breath and your sweat. Even when it is cold you're still sweating, and we weren't able to shower for over a week! Even if we'd had water to wash our clothes with it was so cold they would never have dried, so, as you can imagine, we were all starting to smell really bad!

Finally, after being holed up in the hut for five days, Mr Chou and Mr Kim arrived back with the big camera and Soo Young was carried back up to Kibo. I don't think she was very happy at the prospect of having to climb to the top but she didn't have much choice. That's what she'd been told to do and she just had to get on and do it. In fact the climbing rules stated that if you had to take someone down the mountain for whatever reason then they weren't allowed back up again. Also, you weren't supposed to go up to the summit if you'd had altitude sickness. But the Koreans just ignored those rules and so at five o'clock the next morning I got up and packed a day bag and we all gathered outside to discover it was snowing. Six porters were assigned to look after me and two for Soo Young and off we set. When we weren't filming we sang loudly and 'my boys' as I called them were a lot of fun. It was very steep and slippery but they just kept going, pushing and pulling my wheelchair like a rickshaw. In fact they were so strong that we kept getting ahead of the others and had to stop and wait for them to catch up several times. As usual, when the going got too tough I'd jump out and go up on my backside.

When we got to the Hans Myer Cave all the porters were getting pretty tired and we still had to climb another four or five hours up to Gilman's Point, the second highest peak at 5685 metres. The highest, Uhuru, is another 215 metres (about a two-hour climb) further up. So we did a bit of filming around the cave, which was much smaller than I'd expected, and then Hong Bin and Soo Young and the other climbers set off again with Matt and me and our porters and Mr Kim the cameraman bringing up the rear. By this stage it was getting late in the day, it was snowing and raining and the going was getting steeper and rougher with huge rocks to climb over. We made it to within sight of Gilman's, which was a lot further than many of those who'd passed through Kibo while we were there, but by then I was absolutely knackered. From thereon up it was all steep, foothold stuff requiring ropes and it would have been far too dangerous to have carried on. Staying overnight on the mountain wasn't an option because of the cold temperatures and by this time we'd already been going for over 10 hours. Matt said he was amazed we'd got as far as we had and so we decided at that point to call it quits. We'd done the best we could and it seemed the safest and wisest thing for us to do was to head back to Kibo.

The ironic thing was that I was the healthiest out of the three of us taking part in the documentary yet I was just physically unable to go any further. But as far as I was concerned I'd achieved my goal. I was as close to the top of the mountain as I could get and a lot closer than many of the able-bodied climbers I'd seen attempting the climb. So we began our descent but the Koreans carried on in the most unbelievable conditions. There was snow and sleet and Matt reckoned they were quite mad. He said no New Zealand climber would have even considered doing it, but it just didn't seem to worry them at all. I had never been so cold in my life and I was wet and my muscles ached but we went back down to Kibo a lot faster than we'd gone up! In fact it took us only two hours to get back to the hut and I went most of the way on my backside. It was too dangerous to take me down in my chair and so I was tied by rope to a couple of the porters. I had my heavy-duty plastic pants on and I kept sliding on the ice. Every time I slipped the porters would be slipping too and trying to hold me back. At one place I slipped over 100 metres down the ice. There were huge rocks everywhere so it was pretty dangerous and Matt was a bit unhappy because Elaine had threatened to kill him if I hurt myself. The only way I was able to stop myself was to put my hands in some soft scoria and drag myself to a halt, otherwise I probably wouldn't have stopped till I hit the bottom of the mountain. Maybe I'd have got into the *Guinness Book of Records* for the fastest descent of Kilimanjaro.

Matt made me get back into my rickshaw after that. Ten hours up and two hours down! The others didn't get back to the hut until after ten o'clock that night, cold and covered in ice. It had snowed the whole time and they'd all absolutely had it but they'd made it right to the very top, which was fantastic. I was really glad for them. It must have been treacherous coming down in the dark, though. While we were waiting anxiously for them to return I noted in my diary:

> *The boys did a great job getting me down. I got a flat tyre just as we arrived back at the hut so that will give me something to do later on, fixing it. Did I mention how cold and boring it is here? Most people only stay here one day. This is our fifth. They say that staying at this altitude is not good for you. Anyway, we're going down to the main gate in one hit tomorrow hopefully. I want a hot shower and a good night's sleep. Matt has just gone up the track a bit to see if the others are coming. He's getting a bit concerned as many of them don't have wet-weather gear and it hasn't stopped raining all day. I'm really glad we decided to come down. I don't need to be a hero. I just want to get home now but I have to say this has been a great experience. It is just that we've been here too long. I spend most of my time in my sleeping bag with a balaclava wrapped around my stumps as it gets really cold.*

We had a short celebration once the others got back from the top and then went to bed but my breather had completely packed up by then so I had a restless night and was up again by 5.30 a.m. the next day. We left Kibo at seven o'clock and headed down to Marangu Gate. It was much easier going down because the guys held the front of my chair up and we just powered along. I don't know how my wheelchair stood up to it but the boys were on a mission as it was the tenth and last day. Only problem was it bucketed down with rain all the way. We'd only just got going when it started and it didn't let up. The porters were slipping and sliding all over the place but it just felt so good to finally be going down and back to civilisation!

It was like having a weight taken off our shoulders and we could have put up with anything going down. I'd done many things in my life but climbing Mt Kilimanjaro was definitely the most difficult thing I'd ever experienced. It really was. If anyone asked me whether I'd go back up I'd say, 'No way.' I didn't wake up one morning and think to myself: 'I must climb Mt Kilimanjaro.' It was never a goal of mine. It was just an opportunity that came my way and I'm very glad I had the experience. As far as I know I'm the first person in a wheelchair to get to Gilman's Point. In fact I think there have only been a couple of other people in wheelchairs who've tried climbing 'Kili' and they never got past Kibo, but I think they were far more wheelchair-bound than me. Matt reckoned the guys who built my chair deserved a medal for the way it stood up to the conditions on the mountain. Converting it into a sort of rickshaw was a great idea. Here's an excerpt from my diary about that last day:

> *It was raining most of the day and really slippery. The rocks and steps were really difficult and I wore out three pairs of gloves on the way down trying to brake. We went through Horombo and Manara doing about 30 kilometres an hour. Afterwards I felt like I'd been riding a jetski for eight hours in a 10-foot surf! I was bashed around and tired but elated nevertheless.*

When we got back to the point where the Jeep had dropped us off at the start of the climb we found it waiting for us again because by this stage Soo Young was really quite ill. She wasn't a big girl and I think the physical strain was all too much for her on top of the altitude sickness.

The rest of us were all wet and covered in mud but the relief of having made it back down in one piece was fantastic and no doubt the documentary will show the jubilation on our faces. Seventeen of us squashed into the nine-seater vehicle to go down to Marangu Gate, where we said a sad goodbye to our porters. Next we went to a nearby hotel where Matt and I cleaned my wheelchair and then had the best hot showers we'd ever had in our lives. I don't think I had ever gone ten days without a shower before and it was great to feel clean again. My next priority was to find a phone and ring home and then have some proper food and a decent night's sleep. But, as my diary notes, the last wasn't to be:

> *Monday, 23 December. Only slept half the night as the power went off and I could only snore. Matt reckons he's getting used to it by now. It is a fine morning, no clouds and significantly warmer. What a difference a day and 4000 metres makes. We went back to Marangu Gate this morning to get our certificates for climbing Kilimanjaro and then drove to Arusha for lunch. A Chinese restaurant — surprise, surprise!*

From Arusha we travelled all the way across the border to Nairobi in Kenya. What a journey! I swear there were bugs the size of houses hitting the windscreen of the bus. We had to stop three times to clear it as the driver just couldn't see where he was going. We reached Nairobi at nine o'clock that night and just for something different we went to a Korean restaurant for dinner! Then we booked into the 680 Hotel, which was quite a good place with a lift but no air conditioning. Matt and I were on the ninth floor and Matt reckoned the mosquitoes didn't fly that high. Yeah, right. We both got bitten *all* night! The next day, Christmas Eve, we went out to a farming area to film us meeting with some Masai herdsmen as we had done earlier in the trip in Tanzania. They told me to wear my blue shirt, which I did, but apparently it was the wrong blue shirt. The crew had a half-hour conference about it and in the end decided to do two takes: one with me and one without. Then it was back to Nairobi and another Korean restaurant for dinner. By this stage I was starting to get used to chilli sauce, but I still couldn't believe the way Jeanie put raw chillis and onions on absolutely everything. Even the effects of the chilli sauce weren't enough to protect us from another mozzie attack that night, though!

My diary entry for Christmas Day says it all:

What a place to be on Christmas Day! I talked to everyone at home this morning. Wish I was there with them. So close and yet so far. The streets around the hotel are littered with drunks and derelicts so we decided to stay in our room until lunchtime … three guesses where we ate! We all had a good time, though, and then Matt and I spent the rest of the day in our room reading magazines and watching TV.

The following day we visited a giraffe zoo, which was absolutely amazing. We were filmed feeding the giraffes and they ate out of our hands with their long, slimy tongues. That night we were invited to the Korean Embassy for dinner. It was a magnificent old house and the people were all really pleasant. We enjoyed telling the other guests all about our experiences up Kilimanjaro.

Friday, 27 December was election day in Kenya and a public holiday as that was the only way they could get the people to vote. We were warned there might be demonstrations and riots as the elections are usually rigged, and a truck carrying voting papers had already been hijacked. No one seemed to take much notice of the warning, however, and as it turned out the day passed quite peacefully. We flew out of Nairobi two days later, on the 29th, and landed in Kuala Lumpur the following day, where we stayed the night.

The New Year arrived as we were flying from Kuala Lumpur to Korea and was a complete non-event. I called Elaine before we boarded our plane and she'd already seen in the New Year in New Zealand and gone to bed. At that stage I didn't know when I'd be flying home as Jeanie had said to me just as we were leaving Nairobi: 'I've got some good news and some bad news for you. The good news is that we're going home. The bad news is that we haven't any confirmed flights out of Korea to New Zealand for you and Matt.' Great! Apparently, the only confirmed flight I had was for 10 January. There was no way was I hanging around in Korea a whole week. I'd been away from home a whole month and I just wanted to be reunited with my family. Once we got to Korea, though, we managed to get a flight out again that same night, so Matt and I got a couple of rooms at a hotel near the airport and slept most of the day.

more mountains to climb 9

'Never say never' and 'never give up.'

We arrived back in Auckland from Korea at eleven o'clock on the morning of 2 January 2003. Elaine, Danie, Nikki, Quentin and my two grandsons were all there to meet me, and Houston and Xavier were holding balloons and signs that said 'Welcome Home Pop'. It was a great reunion. Lucas had to work, so he wasn't able to be there but I caught up with him the following week. So we came straight home where another surprise awaited me. In my absence Elaine and my parents and Elaine's dad and friends had got together and painted our swimming pool and landscaped the area around it. The pool is right outside the large floor-to-ceiling window in our lounge and looks out over miles of rolling countryside to the city of Tauranga in the distance. Elaine had covered the garden around it in sand-coloured stones dotted with rocks and ornaments to give it a very Mediterranean ambience. It looked absolutely fantastic. That night my mum and dad and the girls and my grandsons came round for a barbecue and I can't begin to tell you what it was like to have good old Kiwi tucker again. It was bliss being able to tuck into barbecued steak and sausages after all that boiled chicken and rice in Africa. I've warned Elaine I don't want to eat Asian food again for a very long time!

It was wonderful to be back with my family and for the next few weeks we spent most of our time together in the pool. Well, when I was home that is. Within a week of returning from my Kilimanjaro expedition I was back on a plane and winging my way to the United States to address a 1000-strong conference in Miami. I also had speaking engagements in Australia and the South Island of New Zealand. After spending so much time in Africa worrying about my health and whether I'd be fit enough to climb Kilimanjaro, I was involved in two incidents within a fortnight of coming home that could have had far more serious repercussions than any health hazards I'd struck in Tanzania. The first was when I nearly got knocked down on a pedestrian crossing in Miami, and then, about a week after that I had another lucky escape when I suffered my first major mishap during a presentation in Christchurch, New Zealand. I always shin up some trestles and sit on a painter's plank when I'm speaking. As usual, with a New Zealand engagement, I'd organised for a local firm to set up the equipment for me and everything had seemed OK when I checked it. So there I was, up on stage in the middle of my plank, two metres off the ground, talking to an audience of several hundred people when suddenly, without any warning, the whole structure collapsed and I landed very heavily and unexpectedly on the floor. It turned out that the metal trestle poles were very old and rusty and I guess having to support my weight proved too much for them. As I say, I came crashing down onto the stage below, but amazingly only one or two people realised there'd been an accident. The rest all seemed to think it was just part of my act, especially as I managed to recover my composure quickly and continue talking as if nothing had happened. It was only after I'd finished and tried to get back into my wheelchair that I realised I'd actually injured myself and would subsequently need weeks of physiotherapy to come right.

So, having survived Kilimanjaro, Christchurch nearly got the better of me! Thank goodness the accident didn't happen before my trip to Africa. I just wouldn't have been able to go. My arm and shoulder were so sore I could hardly move around the house let alone propel my wheelchair up a mountain. Now I check and double-check my trestles before each show.

My change of course into inspirational speaking all started when a friend, Lawrence O'Toole, asked me to speak to a group of long-term unemployed people who were attending a course he was running in Tauranga. I began going along once a week during their lunch hour to talk to them about the workforce from the point of view of an employer and also the challenges I faced as a double amputee. I did that for a year and thoroughly enjoyed the experience and the feedback I got. Lawrence also asked me to speak to his Rotary group and not long after that I did a motivational course in personal leadership and another in business management. Because of my success both with these courses and also with my own business, I was one of five award winners invited to speak at a special function at the Sheraton Hotel in Auckland.

By this time I was beginning to enjoy public speaking but I'd never heard of professional inspirational speakers until Jim Hainey from Speakers New Zealand approached me and offered to put me on his books. Then author and journalist Paul Smith wrote a chapter about me in his 1997 book *Success in New Zealand Business II*, and I was invited to give a 10-minute talk about my life to the 400 people who attended the book launch. This time Debbie Tawse from Celebrity Speakers New Zealand asked if I was interested in doing some work for her and suddenly I could see a window of opportunity opening up and a new career beckoning.

Around this time a friend asked me if I'd like to go along to the local Toastmasters Club with him one night. I went and listened to different members practising their oratorial skills. Towards the end of the evening they had an activity called Table Topic, where a subject was picked and then a name drawn out of a hat, and that person had to speak on the chosen subject for one minute. That very first night my name was drawn and I was asked to speak for a minute on the subject of kitchen detergents. Now, as Elaine will tell you, that in itself was a bit of a joke. I don't really know a lot about such things because I never do the dishes! The only time I ever tried I put a large amount of ordinary dish-washing liquid into the dishwasher, and we ended up with froth and bubbles floating around the kitchen for two weeks afterwards! Hence I'm not allowed to do the dishes any more. Not a bad trick, huh?

I managed to bluff my way through a minute on the subject of kitchen detergents and at the end of the evening I was presented with a trophy for the best speech. There was a guy sitting next to me who'd apparently been going along to Toastmasters for about six months and we got talking afterwards. He was absolutely amazed that I'd won the trophy on my very first attempt and he seemed genuinely pleased for me.

The next Wednesday night I went along again and sat next to the same guy. We had a little chat and he asked me what I did for a living so I told him I was a signwriter but that I also did a little bit of speaking. When it came to Table Topic time once again my name was drawn out of the hat and I was given a minute to talk on the subject of wooden spoons. Now what the heck do I know about wooden spoons? But I talked for a minute about them anyway, or rather, I used one of the humorous stories from my speaking repertoire and somehow made it end up about wooden spoons, which is a trick you're allowed to use at Toastmasters. At the end of the evening I won the trophy again and the guy sitting beside me just couldn't believe it. 'You've won that trophy two weeks in a row,' he exclaimed. 'Man, that's really amazing.' Somehow I got the impression that this time he wasn't quite so pleased.

Back I went the following week and I can't for the life of me remember what topic I had to talk about this time but I remember the guy beside me also had his name drawn out that night, but once again it was me who won the trophy. This time it was just too much for my newfound friend. He leant across to me and exploded: 'I've been coming here for SIX months now and I haven't won that b... trophy once! How come you've won it three times in a row?' Then he added somewhat suspiciously: 'What did you say you did for a living?' Somehow I couldn't bring myself to tell him I was actually in the process of becoming a professional speaker but after that I decided it was best not to go to Toastmasters again!

I'm working hard at my goal of becoming the best inspirational speaker in the world. I'll know I've really made it when I'm chosen to address meetings in the United States in preference to such well-established speakers as Zig Zigler. He's been one of the top inspirational speakers there for many years. He has a very novel way of speaking both with his country drawl and the message he imparts and he's well respected. So look out Zig Zigler, here I come!

I'm getting an increasing number of engagements in that part of the world. My speaking life is all a far cry from those lunchtime talks I used to give to the unemployed in Tauranga, but it was from those humble beginnings that I realised I had the ability to get up in front of an audience and entertain and, hopefully, inspire people.

I hardly had time to catch my breath last summer. After Miami I had several trips to Australia, umpteen engagements around New Zealand and as I finish this book I've just addressed a huge conference in Singapore. It was the annual Asia and Pacific Life Insurance conference attended by 11,000 people — my biggest audience to date. It was in a huge auditorium with a giant screen on either side of the stage so that those sitting at the back had a better view of the speakers. There were insurance agents from countries such as China, Japan, Vietnam and Thailand, and besides giving the keynote address I also conducted a workshop for 3000 people. People tend to think of workshops as an event where you just sit there and get lectured for an hour or two but mine don't work like that. I like to get everyone involved in a variety of activities to press home my message about attitude, goal setting and making the most of life. For instance, Asian people love karaoke and so

I take one of the songs I've had composed for my presentations and I get them all singing it because the words are so apt and it makes everyone feel good. In Singapore I got everybody up in front of the stage with my trademark cartoon of myself in the background and we all sang along to the song 'Know What I Mean' that Martin Way wrote after he'd read my first book, *Race You to the Top*.

KNOW WHAT I MEAN
Know me, know what's inside your mind, your heart
And see, close your eyes and make a start
The single seed that we sow
And soon the branches will grow
This is make-believe without the dreaming

You can take my hand and climb to the top
Ride stormy waters and you won't want to stop
You can chase all your wishes and capture your dreams
You can do anything you want
If you know what I mean

Mamma said learn how to walk before you run
But I felt the wind in my face
And the joy of much more fun
The river returns to the sea, as the spirit strives to be free
Eyes wide open — so wide you see tomorrow

Chorus:
And there is no need to find — the answer is there inside
If you find you're alone again — understand the words I've said

It was a great way to get everybody warmed up and enjoying themselves and I think that's one of the important things about being an inspirational speaker. You're not just telling a story, you're also enteraining people, and there are all sorts of tools you can use to get your message across in a fun way. I also do a Rolf Harris-type act whereby I sketch a cartoon picture on the computer that's shown up on the big screens. I'll be talking about people's perceptions and at first it looks as if I'm drawing a naked body. A naked woman, in fact. I tell my audience that I was drawing this picture in a public place once when I noticed 10 people gathered around me. I drew a few more strokes and the crowd grew to 20 and then 30 and I couldn't work out why they were all watching me. I go on to talk a bit more about the dangers of people having preconceived ideas and jumping to wrong conclusions and then I finish my drawing and it ends up being a big, floppy-eared dog. It is a more entertaining way of reinforcing my point.

Another gimmick I use in my workshops to show how people see and hear things in different ways is to write out a message on a piece of paper and give to someone at the back of the room, a version of 'Chinese Whispers'. They have to then tell it to the person in front of them, who relays it to someone in front of them and so it goes on until the message arrives on the front row. I invariably find it is completely different to the original message I wrote on the piece of paper. Again it is all about people's perceptions: how they hear and see things. Students are often asked to explain what an author was trying to say in a certain book and so they write a synopsis only to discover that they've lost the plot completely. Pity the police when they're conducting an investigation into a serious accident or incident. They must get so frustrated, not to mention confused, by the different eye-witness accounts they're given. While one person will give a categorical description of the make of an offender's car, the colour, the age, who was driving it and where and when the incident happened, someone else will be equally confident in giving a completely different set of facts. Because so many of us just see what we want to see. I once read that half the people who complain to the Broadcasting Authority about something they've supposedly seen or heard on television or radio didn't actually see or hear it themselves. They heard about it second or third hand and in the process quite often got the wrong end of the stick.

These days some people stare at me not just because I'm in a wheelchair but also because they've been to one of my presentations or else they've seen me on television or in the newspaper. Just recently, when Elaine and I went down to the Tauranga waterfront to look at the boats that had stopped over during the Around Alone yacht race we overheard a guy telling his friends about me. He said: 'Oh, look, there's Tony Christiansen. He's just climbed Mt Fujiama.' Now Mt Fuji happens to be in Japan and that's a country I haven't visited since I was sixteen. But, hey, he'd got half the story right! And that's what so many people do, they only get half the story right because they only see or hear what they want to.

When I'm a keynote speaker at a conference I like to break my presentation up a bit by showing two-and-a-half minute video clips of some of my sporting activities, such as skydiving, white-water rafting, motor racing and flying a plane. In future I'll also be able to add clips from the Mt Kilimanjaro documentary as well as film of me scuba diving. And I also like to play the songs I've had written for me because I think the words are so very apt.

My presentations have changed over the years as I've become more experienced and confident and achieved more goals. These days I make more use of technology and computer graphics and I also pick up little tips from watching and listening to other speakers.

In order to become the best inspirational speaker in the world I really need to become better known in the United States, and to that end I'd really love to spend some time there in the not too distant future. I dream of Elaine and me getting a mobile home or RV (Recreational Vehicle), as they call it over there, and spending a few months touring around the States. I love America. It is such a vast country and there's so much to do and see. All that motor racing and all those air shows! I'd be in my element. While there I would like to try and get my name better known on the speaking circuit. I really enjoy addressing larger groups of people these days and they have some huge corporate conferences in the States. And one thing about Americans is that they love the underdog. They love to see people who have challenges in their lives go out there and succeed. Look how they idolise basketball stars such as Michael Jordan, Shaquille O'Neal and others like them who rose up from the ghettos to become the best and highest paid at their chosen sport. They celebrate that sort of success in the United States. That's one of the things I really love about Americans and it is a concept we really struggle with here in New Zealand. We're too busy trying to knock people down and bring them down a level rather than encouraging them and inspiring them to go to greater heights. I think that's an attitude New Zealanders really have to work on. It is one of the many challenges we face as a nation.

After living in New Zealand for 44 years I wouldn't mind doing something different with my life and perhaps try living in either the United States or Australia for six months of the year and spend the other six months at home in Tauranga. It is just a thought. A dream maybe. The past three years have brought a dramatic change in lifestyle for Elaine and me. We have our beautiful new home and we get to travel to exotic places and do exciting and adventurous things. Who knows what the next three years will bring? There are still heaps of things I'd like to have a go at. I was watching a TV programme about hydroplanes recently and I thought, 'Yes, that's me, that's me.' I get very excited watching sports like that. All that horsepower! I wouldn't mind having a go at drag racing some time too.

I don't know whether I'll actually ever get around to these things but it is great to know that I've got that choice, that I've got the ability to make it happen if I want it to. We only get one chance at life and I'm not about to waste it. I want my brief time here on Earth to count for something when I've gone. Hopefully, 10, 20 or maybe 50 years after I've departed this life someone will read one of my books or watch one of the documentaries I've been in and say, 'Wow, that guy Tony Christiansen sure knew how to get the most out of life!'

As I write this book there's a chance I might be taking part in the Sydney-Hobart yacht race in December. A woman approached me after a presentation I gave in Sydney recently and suggested I get in touch with an organisation over there called Disabled Sailing in Australia. Apparently a group of disabled yachties always takes part in the prestigious annual event and so I've emailed them to say I'd be interested in joining the crew. It is another opportunity that has presented itself, like climbing Kilimanjaro. The race is a huge event in Australia and can be quite treacherous at times, which is why I haven't told Elaine about it yet! She'll find out when she reads this book. It would also mean another Christmas away from home, so I guess I'll have to give it some serious thought before I make a commitment. But whether I get to sail in it or not doesn't really matter. It is the fact that the opportunity has arisen that's the exciting part.

Another idea that's been mooted in recent times is the possibility of having my own television show. Again, that's something I'd love to be involved with. I'd love a show whereby I helped people overcome their fear of attempting adventurous feats such as white-water rafting or flying or skydiving. I could take someone who was afraid of heights out for a tandem skydive, for instance, or if they were afraid of flying I could take them up in a light plane. Although, on second thoughts, I'm not sure just how much the sight of a pilot with no legs would help allay their fears! I'd love to be involved in a programme like that because it would be another way of getting my message across. It is fine to write a book and share your story that way or to talk about it on stage, but there are so many people who talk about things and don't actually do them. I'd really like to be able to show people what they can achieve if they put their mind to it, and prove to them that they can take risks, pursue goals and make dreams come true. It would be another opportunity for me to experience new things as well.

Who knows, perhaps one day someone will even make a movie about me? That's what's about to happen to Colin Meads. Well, when I say about to happen, he reckons it has been in the negotiation stage for about four years now, but as I write this he thinks they might finally be getting close to choosing the cast. News of the planned movie first hit the headlines last year at a time when Colin says he was 'fortunately out of the country'. As a result Verna had to field the phone calls from the media and so when asked who she thought should play the roles of herself and Colin she rattled off the first film stars she could think of — Sandra Bullock and Ben Affleck. Colin seems quite bemused by the whole idea and, like me, he's constantly amazed at the opportunities that present themselves in life, be they big ones like the movie, or smaller happenings like the one he relates here:

'I went to see my 15-year-old grandson, Clinton, taking part in the school rowing championships on Lake Karapiro recently and one of the organisers asked if I'd be back for the finals a couple of days later. I said I was hoping to get back from Wellington in time to see my grandson row in the finals and he said: "Oh well, if you're here for the prize-giving we'll get you to present some of the prizes." Now, I'm a guy who knows absolutely nothing about rowing. That was the first time I'd ever watched it other than on television during the Olympic Games. And suddenly here I am, being asked to present prizes to these school kids. In many ways it is quite nice but I still think it is a bit unusual for someone who knows nothing about the sport to be doing the honours! But as Tony says, it is amazing how many things happen like that, just out of the blue. I've got 14 grandchildren, three grandsons and 11 granddaughters, and they're all interested in their respective sports. Verna and I try to watch them as often as we can at

weekends, although I must admit Verna does the rounds more than I do. But I often go to netball because my granddaughters get round me by pleading: 'Come on, Grandad, you've got to come and watch us play.' I was still playing rugby when my own children were growing up and like a lot of fathers I was always busy and I guess I never spent enough time with them. But you seem to have more time later in life for your grandchildren and we're fortunate that they all live fairly close, either in Hamilton or Te Kuiti.'

Life is certainly never dull for Colin Meads and you don't have to be good at rugby to take a page or two out of his book. Like so many high-achievers he set himself goals and worked hard to get where he is today. Find something you're good at or that you enjoy doing, and give it all you've got. You may not end up as well known as Colin Meads, but you'll be a happier, more fulfilled person and you may surprise yourself with what you can achieve.

Because I have a flair for public speaking and I'm never too shy to voice my opinions on life, it is often been suggested I should take up politics as a profession. Who knows, perhaps I will one day. But I always reckon that if I was to enter either local government or national politics I'd have to be Mayor or Prime Minister! I could never settle for just being a councillor or an ordinary Member of Parliament. I'd want to be able to make a big difference. To be truthful I haven't got the patience to be a politician.

It all boils down to making sure that whatever you choose to do, you do to the best of your ability. As I've said many times before, life is over in the flick of an eyelid, so you owe it yourself to make every second count.

I believe life is like a row of three boxes. The first is a little box in the middle that contains all the things we *know* we know. That's our own comfortable life that we know all about. On one side is a slightly larger box that contains the things we know we *don't know*. For instance, I know a little bit about a lot of different sports but I don't know how to play them all. I can name a lot of wild animals but I can't tell you all about their habitats and eating habits. I meet a lot of people through my speaking engagements but I don't know *all* about them. Then there's the third box. It is a huge one that contains all the things we *don't know* we don't know. There are so many things in the universe that I have absolutely no idea about. There are millions of stars and planets I know nothing about. New sea creatures are being found every day in the oceans around the world, and in places like New Guinea, for instance, they're finding animals even the scientists have never seen or heard of before. Compared with the contents of that huge box, our lives here on Earth represent such a tiny moment in time, like a grain of sand on the beach. But we all want our grain of sand or our moment in time to actually mean something so that we're not just here today and gone tomorrow. In our hearts each and every one of us wants to leave a legacy so that our life has had a purpose even if it is just bringing up our children to be worthy citizens or being the best mother, father, sister or son that we could possibly be. When you consider the big box of things we *don't know we don't know* we really are here for such a brief moment in time. So many people have wasted that moment when in fact they've had the opportunity to do something with it. It is what you do with your time that counts but so many people are existing in this revolving spiral whereby they get up in the morning, go to work, come home and go to bed and that's it. They don't have the inclination or the courage or the wisdom to look for opportunities and take risks and dream of ways to do more with their lives.

That's why I get such a kick out of some of the letters and emails I get from people who've read my books or heard me speak. It is one thing to address a big conference like the one in Singapore where 11,000 people all clap and cheer when they hear about my achievements but it is so much more special to get a personal message from someone whose life I have touched. For instance, out of the blue I got an email from a guy who used to work at our local service station. He asked if I remembered him and I did indeed. I'd seen him there many times and one day a couple of years ago I was at the pumps when he came running out full of excitement and said he'd just bought my book and started reading it and he thought it was great. The next time I stopped for petrol he'd brought the book to work and he got me to sign it for him. Shortly after that he left and I didn't see or hear from him for over a year. His email said that after reading my book he'd been inspired to pursue his dream of being a teacher and that he was currently at training college and doing really well. He said he'd read my book several times and now keeps it by his bed so he can pick it up and refer to it occasionally. He said that he'd gone through periods of depression and reading my book was the only thing that had pulled him through. Elaine and I love getting feedback like that because it shows that I'm getting my message across and making a difference in people's lives.

My professional life now involves encouraging people to think a little bit differently about themselves and the opportunities they have. To think positively and strive to achieve their goals. I don't presume to try and sort out people's individual personal problems. What I can do, though, is offer advice on how to overcome a broad spectrum of challenges that each one of us is confronted with at some time in our lives. I want to help people create a better environment for themselves, be it at work or at home, by offering some simple suggestions for them to think about. I want to inspire them to think about *what* they want to do, *why* they want to do it and *how* they're going to do it. So often when you ask someone what it is they want out of life they can't tell you. They just don't know. How on earth can you make any goals to work towards if you don't know what it is you want in the first place?

I always maintain there are three types of people in the world: those who are making things happen, those who want to make things happen and those who are wondering *what the hell happened?* Which one are you? It is up to you to decide which you want to be. But you can only blame yourself if you're sitting there wondering what the heck happened as the world rushes by because nothing ever stays the same.

The people who want things to happen have set themselves goals and they're working to achieve them. As for the people who are actually making things happen, they're the ones who are already out there taking the chances, putting the money up and enjoying the success. People call them lucky but more often than not they've got where they are today by courage, determination, self-motivation and sheer hard slog. But they too started off with simple dreams and goals. My goal is to inspire people to dream dreams and then have the confidence to get stuck in and make those dreams come true. I'd like to think that by sharing my experiences and thoughts on life I can make a difference to other people's lives and I've certainly been encouraged and grateful for the feedback I've had so far.

In spite of my ambition to be the best inspirational speaker in the world and despite all my sporting interests, at the end of the day the thing that gives me the greatest satisfaction and pleasure is to be at home watching my grandsons play in the swimming pool. To me it is the best money I've ever spent because of the sheer enjoyment I get from being with them and watching them enjoy it. Houston's been learning to swim and since we built the pool his confidence has increased in leaps and bounds.

So here I am, at 44 years of age with a means of earning money that's more than just a job; it is a passion and I love every minute of it. I get to travel to some extraordinary places and meet so many great people and then I can return to Tauranga and enjoy my home comforts. Now, how wonderful is that? How much better than just sitting around in my wheelchair wishing I had my legs back so I could be 'normal'?

As I finish this book I've just returned from nine nights away, flying all over the country and backwards and forwards to Australia several times on speaking engagements. Sometimes Elaine and I are like ships that meet in the night. But now I'm taking a whole week off and we're going up north to Tutukaka so that I can hopefully unwind a little and do some diving. Next month we're off to Orlando in Florida. Winter is a busy time for me because many big businesses like to take their staff away to some warm, exotic location such as Fiji, Vanuatu or the Gold Coast of Australia to revitalise and remotivate them.

So before I throw my wetsuit and weights into my van let me remind you of some things that I believe to be true:

- ~ We don't know what the future holds, so try living for the moment.
- ~ Don't harbour grudges and regrets.
- ~ Get rid of all that excess negative baggage.
- ~ You can only have one thought at a time and it is either going to be positive or negative. Train yourself to always think positively.
- ~ Make the most of every opportunity that comes your way.
- ~ Have your dreams and your goals for tomorrow, but don't waste a minute of today.
- ~ You achieve success by choice and not by chance. Life is full of choices so make sure you choose well.
- ~ Don't let anybody take your dreams away from you.
- ~ Never, ever say 'never'. Don't let people tell you what you can't do.
- ~ As Martin wrote in the song that follows, never give up.

NEVER GIVE UP

Though life can be a battle
You take things as they come
Though the mirror might be shattered
You know the race is never won
When you look into the faces
And the eyes don't seem the same
Is it the reason that you play the game?

When you reach atop the mountain
Which horizon do you see?
Or are the hazy skies upon you
And you're frightened just to be?
Are you scared to ride the dragon
As he climbs into the sun?
Are you prepared?
Your life has just begun.

I can see tomorrow, though the road has its turn
We can be there tomorrow, depending what we learn

Never give up on love
Never give up on your destiny or prayers from above
Never give up, though hopeless it seems
No, never give up on your dreams

If I had the wings I'd fly for you
Chase the moon into the night
And I know sometimes you think you're dealt
A hand that isn't right
You can remember where you've been

But keep your eyes always ahead
You can remember that I'm always there

I can see tomorrow though the bridges may burn
We can be there tomorrow, depending what we learn